HEALTHY PREGNANCY
THE YOGA WAY

HEALTHY PREGNANCY
THE YOGA WAY

Judi Thompson

Foreword by
James C. Baker, M.D.

Photographs by
FRANK L. FEISTAL

Dolphin Books
Doubleday & Company, Inc.
Garden City, N.Y.
1977

Library of Congress Cataloging in Publication Data

Thompson, Judi.
Healthy pregnancy the yoga way.

"A Dolphin original."
1. Pregnancy.   2. Prenatal care.   3. Yoga,
Hatha.   I. Title.   [DNLM: 1. Pregnancy—Popular
works.   2. Yoga.   WQ150 T473h]
RG525.T49   618.2′4

A Dolphin Original

ISBN: 0-385-11631-4
Library of Congress Catalog Card Number 76–23818

First Edition

To Bikram
Who made it all possible

ACKNOWLEDGMENTS

My sincere thanks to:

James C. Baker, M.D.
Dr. William A. Cook, M.D.
Robert B. Stone
Leta Laborde
Ananda
Linda County
Malia Black
Susana Sori
Susan D. Chung, R.N.
Mrs. R. Keehnel, R.N.
Maria Rosenstein
E. Claybrook
Joy Gardiner

With deep appreciation to my parents, Cdr. William P. Blackmore and Jean Blackmore, for their continuing help and support and to my children, Terri Anne Kailani, David, Rebecca, and Michael Jai.

A special note of appreciation to Millie Jue Tsui, assistant library specialist, Hamilton Library, University of Hawaii, for generously sharing her expertise in bibliographic research methods and her extensive and thorough knowledge of library resources.

Photography by Frank L. Feistal, Camera Graphics, Inc., Honolulu, Hawaii.

CONTENTS

FOREWORD

The creation of an entirely new being within a woman is truly a beautiful and wondrous phenomenon, and a healthy, happy pregnancy culminating in a joyous childbirth experience is the normal wish of every expectant mother. Judi Blackmore Thompson, a teacher of Yoga and four times a mother herself, presents a clear and thorough explanation of the significant role Yoga can play in maternal health. She has personally practiced the self-discipline and exercises fundamental to Yoga and recommends them with enthusiasm and the sincere wish that her readers benefit from the practice of Yoga in pregnancy.

I have known Judi and her parents, retired Navy Commander and Mrs. W. P. Blackmore, for more than twenty years; they are among the finest people I know. Judi is an extremely conscientious person of outstanding character and integrity. It is evident that the information she presents in her book has been carefully researched and compiled with a genuine concern for both physical and mental maternal health and happiness.

I recommend this book as worthwhile and rewarding reading, significantly beneficial to prenatal and postnatal maternal health.

JAMES C. BAKER, M.D.
September 1976

CHAPTER

1

YOGA AND PREGNANCY

Why Yoga for Expectant Mothers?

Pregnancy is a unique time in a woman's life and should be experienced as the beautiful and fulfilling condition that it is. Pregnancy is a time of preparation and waiting, but also a time complete unto itself, a time to center yourself, to go within, and to reflect upon the miracle of childbirth. Nothing else can compare to having a baby! All other activities pale in comparison when viewed in the proper perspective. And no one else in the world can have *your* baby.

During pregnancy, a woman undergoes many physical, emotional, and metabolic changes, and her attitudes and feelings toward her pregnancy largely determine her experience. Good health and serenity are particularly vital during this time and bear a direct relationship to the new life developing within. Statistics show that women who live serene and tranquil lives are better able to give birth to healthy children than women burdened with emotional upsets and adjustments, and it is a known fact that people who are emotionally stable are able to retain more of the nutrients they eat than those who are unstable. Emotional disturbances may also result in a decrease in calcium retention, which naturally affects the unborn child.

Pregnancy is the perfect time in which to practice Yoga. These slow-motion exercises from India relieve tension, strengthen and stimulate vital muscles, organs, and glands, and conserve rather than dissipate energy. Through the performance of Yogasanas, muscles are stretched, strengthened, and firmed while the joints utilized in the birth process become flexible. There is no strain or enervating exercise involved in performing the Asanas (postures) of Hatha Yoga. On the contrary, a feeling of peace and well-being accompany the natural relaxation and energization following the performance of Yoga. Concentration and self-control are also enhanced through regular practice of Yoga, as body and mind are integrated and better able to function under full power.

1

Hatha Yoga includes a system of Asanas that concentrates on exercising the spine and awakening the life-force or energy flow within. The word Yoga is derived from the Sanskrit root "yuj," which means join or union. Hatha means the natural harmony of opposites, such as the sun (Ha) and the moon (Tha). This ancient system was designed to restore the inherent balance and harmony of the body within itself. While most systems of exercise, such as calisthenics, utilize vigorous action and emphasize the movement and rhythmic contractions of the muscles, Hatha Yoga is centered on the subtle activity of relaxation into fixed postures without strain or fatigue, and the awakening of the life-energy through simple controlled breathing techniques. This system is beautifully adapted to pregnancy.

Relaxation, a Must!

The ability to relax at will is particularly important during the months before childbirth and is an essential part of an efficient labor. Relaxation is necessary to relieve tension, both of body and of mind. Almost everyone has had the experience of being told to "Relax!" while sitting in a dentist's chair. The automatic response, of course, is not to relax but to stiffen and tighten all the muscles in preparation for the dentist's drill. Tension is the spontaneous reaction to threat of pain as we automatically brace ourselves for what is to come, when what we ought to do is exactly the opposite—relax as completely as possible. Tension is a major cause of pain, and one of the best ways to combat pain is to relax and flow with it. Prepared-childbirth classes teach relaxation techniques to apply to the contractions experienced during labor and delivery. Fear is closely allied to tension in producing pain: By learning what to expect during childbirth, fear is allayed and the possibility of pain further decreased.

Energize as You Relax

Yoga does not tire the body as do strenuous physical exercises. Quite the contrary, as the practice of Yoga renews and energizes the body. The ancient Yogis claimed that the body is a reservoir of infinite strength and life-energy that can be commanded for use by the power of the conscious will. Yoga supplements and completes other systems of exercise, not through outward or mechanical means, but through force of ordinary will power. These classic Yogasanas were conceived thousands of years ago to awaken the life-energy through the tensing of certain muscles in specific postures. These postures are held for a set length of time and immediately followed by complete relaxation for the same length of time as the posture is held. Unless the Asanas are immediately followed by this relaxation, which is an integral part of the posture, the benefits of the pose are negated. It is through this process of tension plus relaxation that the body is energized in a completely natural and healthful way. In order for perfect physical relaxation to occur, however, the tension should be of maximum exertion *without strain*.

In order to attain complete relaxation, you must learn to relax the mind as well as the body. Banish all worries, problems, and negativity for a little while. Learn to "tune out" those thoughts that are bothersome or unsettling. Attune your mind to a scene of beauty or an uplifting thought; or empty your mind of thoughts entirely for complete peace. The ancient practice of meditation is becoming a widespread method of easing mental tensions.

Meditation

It isn't necessary to spend a lot of money to learn how to meditate. Meditation is simply the process of stilling the mind. Practice consists of quietly paying attention, in a calm and contemplative state, to your inner self. The currently popular Transcendental Meditation is a form of mantra Yoga, which seeks to allow the mind to "transcend" the subtlest activity of thinking and reach a state of pure awareness in the source of thought. Another direct form of meditation is to sit upright in a cross-legged position, or in a straight-backed chair if this is more comfortable for you (it is important that the spine remain erect), close your eyes, take several deep breaths, exhaling completely, and "let go." Allow your thoughts to rise like bubbles and watch them come and go, without judgment or attachment to them. Simply observe the thought process until it becomes quiet; then let it be. A quiet mind is a relaxed mind, and meditation is a pleasant and renewing process that is most soothing to the self.

Scientific studies of the meditative process have discovered that definite physical occurrences accompany meditation. Meditators' metabolic rates were reduced by an average of 20 per cent, although blood analysis showed that a normal balance of oxygen to carbon dioxide was maintained. Skin resistance increased, and EEGs of brain waves showed specific changes in certain frequencies wherein Alpha brain waves predominated; these are the brain waves that run from 8 to 13 cycles per second and appear to be related to creativity and a relaxed yet alert mental state. These waves were regular and stronger in amplitude than usual, and in a few cases, low-voltage Alpha brain waves and trains of even slower Theta waves appeared.

If you desire to practice meditation, a perfect time to meditate is immediately following your Yoga practice, as the two disciplines go hand in hand.

Exercise for Two

Everything you do during your pregnancy affects your baby either directly or indirectly as the baby's systematic needs are completely dependent upon the mother's overall health. The body has an increased need for efficient exercise without strain during pregnancy. Yoga exercises are a non-mechanical, completely natural means for strengthening all living tissues and muscle fibers, for accelerating involuntary functions, such as those of the heart, lungs, stomach, and intestines, as well as capillaries, veins, and glands, and to keep them at peak performance without exhausting or overworking them. The awakened life-force, energy, serenity, and peace of mind that are a direct result of regular Yoga practice benefit your baby at the same time they benefit you.

The Importance of Breath

Breathing is the most important of all bodily functions. You can live for quite a while without food or even water, but you can last only a few minutes without oxygen. Oxygen nourishes every cell in the body with life-giving energy and supplies your growing baby with the vitality he needs for maximum development. During labor, it is especially important that the blood flow provides sufficient oxygen for the uterus and that it carries the waste material from the laboring muscles. These waste products, called metabolites, irritate blood vessel walls and muscle fibers when found in high concentration, and if allowed to remain in the body, cause pain. Without a sufficient oxygen supply and the efficient disposal of those metabolites, the abdominal, uterine, and pelvic muscles become tired and overworked, again intensifying pain and prolonging labor.

Learn to breathe deeply, expanding your lungs to their full capacity for increased health and energy. Deep breathing is essential to full relaxation and relief of nervous tension. Keep your rooms well-ventilated with fresh air and proper circulation, and make it a point to get outside in the fresh air at least once a day. A daily walk is not only a pleasant habit to develop during pregnancy, but it is also good exercise for those muscles involved in delivery.

Emotional Changes of Pregnancy

According to a recent study undertaken by Dr. Olive Rich, nursing professor at the University of Pittsburgh, and her staff, an expectant mother's feelings, thoughts and emotions reflected her physical changes during pregnancy.

Most of the women interviewed admitted that they were surprised and not very happy to learn that they were pregnant; some were even annoyed at what they viewed as an interruption in the routine of their lives. Mental anxiety, worries about labor, childbirth, the new baby, and the mother's role accompanied the physical changes during the first part of pregnancy. As pregnancy progressed and physical discomfort grew, feelings centered on hostility toward a cumbersome body, further anxiety, boredom, and the feeling that this process would never end. Worries about the possible abnormality of the baby and of what might go wrong during delivery occurred. Immediately after birth, according to the study, patients reached a state of euphoria and were elated to give birth to a healthy baby after months of living with an unwieldy body. This feeling of happiness was followed by a period of difficulty during the post-partum interval while the mother was still weak and fatigued and beginning to feel trapped and frustrated.

Attitude during pregnancy largely determines the happiness of the experience. A joyful and expectant mental outlook will minimize the minor irritations and discomforts of pregnancy. A woman who is consciously or subconsciously unwilling and fearful of the many changes a baby will bring, will naturally be distressed over many of the changes during pregnancy. A mother who sincerely welcomes her new baby with love and eager anticipation is well on the way to a happy and successful pregnancy and a joyous birth.

Minimizing the Post-partum Blues

The post-partum period is a critical time in developing a sound relationship between mother and child and can be a difficult time for the new mother, who has had a tremendous physical and emotional experience. She is still weak and may feel some discomfort, as her body is not yet back to normal. She may feel irritable and fatigued and nowadays is most likely to be without the extended family help that was the case fifty years ago. She is likely to feel frustrated and angry and then guilty for having these feelings. If she is breast feeding, she is undergoing further changes and discomforts. The professional term used to describe this emotional state is the "post-partum blues."

A new mother doesn't have to experience these post-partum blues. Being *aware* of the condition is preparation in itself. Rest frequently, as soon as you feel fatigue, and stay off of your feet as much as possible. Limit the number of visitors you receive during the first few weeks to immediate family and very close friends, and limit even these visits to twenty minutes. Let the house go; discipline yourself to tune out housework that doesn't need to be attended to immediately. An understanding husband and family can be of enormous help during this time. If they don't happen to be understanding, ignore them! Taking care of yourself and a new baby is a full-time job during the first few weeks after delivery. The dishes will always be there to be done, and housework can wait. This is a time of priorities, and you and your baby are first on the list!

Exercising during this period with the Asanas recommended for the postpartum period is a real help in feeling physically stronger and will be reflected in an improved mental state. Do at least a few Yogasanas daily, even when you don't feel like exercising; this is when you are likely to benefit the most. Breathing exercises and Pranayama techniques play an important part during the post-natal period; you can often lift a blue mood by simply supplying your system with more oxygen!

Eating the right foods also affects the system; energizing natural foods and satisfying, but simple to prepare, menus are best. Keep plenty of natural snack foods on hand for quick energy and a natural boost when fatigue sets in: dried apricots and fruits, raisins and dates, nuts and seeds, fresh fruits and cheese are delicious and pick you up without letting you down a few minutes later. Drinking plenty of fluids is vital during this time, especially if you are a nursing mother. Drink water several times during the day and indulge yourself in all of the fresh fruit and vegetable juices you desire. Coffee, tea, and herb teas in moderation are also a good fluid source.

Yoga and Prepared Childbirth

Prepared-childbirth methods are considered "prepared" rather than "natural" since the mother-to-be is educated beforehand as to the entire birth process and conditioned to respond in a specific matter to specific stimuli (the uterine contraction) through relaxation and breathing techniques. In this way, she is prepared for the soon-to-be experienced labor. In the course of this preparation, the expectant mother develops control of her body. Through the discipline of daily practice, she learns to co-ordinate both mind and body, very much like the person who practices Yoga. Yoga and prepared-childbirth courses, therefore, have much in common as both disciplines enable the mother-to-be truly to know and be in touch with her own mind and body, and are extremely complementary.

The exercises taught in prepared-childbirth courses are simple general exercises concentrating on the lower-abdominal and perineal muscles (the muscles used in labor), leg muscles (to help prevent muscle cramps when legs are in stirrups for delivery), and upper-arm muscles (used in pulling on the handgrips while pushing on the delivery table). Women who have practiced

Yoga find the transition to prepared-childbirth methods extremely easy, while women who have not exercised much sometimes find even a simple leg lift difficult. Women who have studied Yoga and enter prepared-childbirth classes generally remark on the great similarities between the two.

Relaxation is one of the most important learned responses in prepared-childbirth teachings. The normal spontaneous reaction to threat of pain is tension, and it is this very tension that causes pain. It takes much training and bodily control to enable a person to relax on command. Yoga, as a discipline, emphasizes the awareness of the body and bodily functions and trains a person to control them. This training is instrumental in controlled relaxation. A woman who has had both Yoga and prepared-childbirth training should be able to relax quite readily.

The ability to concentrate is a direct by-product of Yoga practice. This ability is also highly important when practicing prepared-childbirth methods and is a necessity in practicing mind-body control.

Prepared-childbirth classes accept expectant mothers from six to eight weeks before their due date—too late to start classes in *both* Yoga and prepared childbirth. It would be ideal if a woman began to study Yoga for pregnant women as soon as she knew she was expecting. That way she would be in good physical condition when she came to prepared-childbirth class, at about seven months gestation, and already trained in relaxation methods, Pranayama techniques, and body control. Although the information specific to childbirth given in the course would be new and would require added practice, the transition into prepared-childbirth methods would be much easier for her, and her experience in Yoga should enable it to be even more meaningful and applicable to the labor and delivery process.

CHAPTER 2

DO'S AND DON'TS DURING PREGNANCY

BASIC RULES
FOR THE MOTHER-TO-BE TO REMEMBER

DON'T STRAIN!

This is the Number One Rule to remember. Each pregnancy is as unique as the woman experiencing it. Your body will tell you what is right for you; listen to it.

DO CONSULT YOUR DOCTOR

The dietary and other recommendations regarding general health and well-being presented in this book have been gathered with conscientious concern for completeness and accuracy. It is not possible in a book this size, however, to provide unlimited counsel covering every aspect of every pregnancy. Therefore, as a routine precaution against unusual medical problems in pregnancy, do consullt your physician for appropriate physical examinations and monitoring. As a general rule, you should also check with your physician before undertaking any exercise program more active than one you may be following at present. Keep in mind that your doctor is the one best qualified to judge what is best for you and your baby.

DON'T WEAR SHOES OR SOCKS WHILE EXERCISING

Bare feet are definitely in order while doing Yoga as classic Yogasanas are traditionally performed barefoot. Not only is it more comfortable for assuming the postures, but it is safer as well; shoes and socks are awkward and slippery.

DO WEAR COMFORTABLE CLOTHING

Loose clothes or leotards are appropriate wear. If you are uncomfortable in a pair of leotards during pregnancy, top them off with a sleeveless top or apron. However, many people feel that a pregnant woman is the most beautiful sight in the world! Why not enjoy it?

DO USE A FIRM MAT

A folded blanket, a thick rug or a foam rubber or exercise mat is appropriate. A pillow or two or a folded towel under your head and legs may help you to perform prone postures more comfortably during the latter months of pregnancy. (See "Savasana.")

DON'T DO SIT-UPS

Never do regular sit-ups from flat on your back during pregnancy. Always roll to one side and push up with the opposite hand to avoid strain.

DO SIT UP PROPERLY

It is important to sit up during pregnancy in such a way as to avoid any strain upon the abdomen, especially after the fifth month. This is achieved from a prone position by rolling to one side and pushing up with the opposite hand absorbing most of the pressure. It is a good idea to get into the habit of rising from any prone position in this manner as soon as you know you are pregnant. You should even get out of bed in the morning this way!

DON'T DO STRENUOUS UPWARD-STRETCHING
OR FORWARD-BENDING POSTURES IN SITTING POSITIONS

However, stretching postures done with mild movements and most standing forward-bending postures are completely safe and help the spine to become strong and elastic.

DON'T DO FACE-DOWN POSTURES

All Asanas that result in pressure on the abdomen are to be avoided.

DON'T DO INVERTED POSTURES

These are not recommended during pregnancy after the third month as the position of the baby may be adversely affected.

DON'T DO UDDIYANA-BANDHA OR OTHER POSTURES INVOLVING VIOLENT STOMACH CONTRACTIONS

Any postures that could adversely affect your baby are to be avoided, of course.

DO CROSS-LEGGED POSTURES

All cross-legged postures are beneficial to pregnant women. These poses help to loosen the knees and hip joints, while stretching the muscles of the pelvic floor and inside thigh. In India, mastery of the Lotus position is said to facilitate painless childbirth.

DO SQUATTING POSTURES

Squatting poses are excellent in helping to develop many of the muscles used in delivery.

DO USE COMMON SENSE

Certain Asanas by their very nature are forbidden during pregnancy after the third month. Other Asanas may become uncomfortable to perform during the latter months of pregnancy. This is an individual matter, and each mother-to-be must adjust her exercise schedule to accommodate her own needs.

DON'T NEGLECT YOUR DIET

Remember that your baby's health depends a great deal upon what you eat. Your diet is his diet, and he is depending on you for the nutrients he needs.

DO CUT DOWN ON COFFEE AND TEA

It is not necessary to eliminate coffee and tea from your diet if you enjoy them, but try to avoid drinking these beverages to excess. Substitute fresh fruit and vegetable juices and healthful herb teas instead.

DO AVOID ALCOHOL AND DRUGS

Although most doctors agree that alcohol in moderation during pregnancy is all right, studies have shown that alcohol is filtered through the liver and can lead to malfunctioning. Do remember that alcohol does enter the bloodstream and does cross the placenta. *Any* drug can affect the system of a pregnant woman adversely (even aspirin) and is a *potential* threat to her unborn child. Unless prescribed by your doctor as necessary, it is best to avoid drugs completely. (See "A Special Warning to Expectant Mothers.")

DO PRACTICE YOGA OUT OF DOORS OR IN A WELL-VENTILATED ROOM

When exercising indoors, open windows to allow as much fresh air as possible to circulate throughout the room.

DON'T PRACTICE YOGA ON A FULL STOMACH

Wait at least an hour after eating before exercising.

DON'T WORRY IF YOU ARE NOT ABLE TO PERFORM EACH ASANA PERFECTLY

It does not matter whether or not you are able to perform each posture exactly as pictured; the exercise will still "work." You are getting as much benefit from performing the pose to the best of your ability as is someone who is able to execute it perfectly.

DO MOVE SLOWLY

Never force the body into postures. Avoid putting stress on your muscles; the body should relax into the Asanas.

DO CLEAR YOUR MIND COMPLETELY

Banish all problems and unhappy thoughts during Yoga practice, forget your worries and concentrate only on the Asanas for maximum benefit.

DO ADAPT YOUR OWN YOGA SCHEDULE

The Asanas given in this book are intended to be used as a guide. Each mother-to-be should adapt her own program to suit her individual needs, with her doctor's consent. Feel free to omit Asanas or parts of Asanas that might cause strain or are uncomfortable to perform. Work within the framework of your own body to develop a schedule of Yogasanas to strengthen, energize, and revitalize yourself in preparation for the exciting times ahead!

DO END YOGA PRACTICE
WITH KAPALBHATI FOLLOWED BY SAVASANA

Always finish your exercise period with Kapalbhati in Vajrasana (Blowing in Fixed Firm Pose) followed by Savasana (Sponge Pose).

A SPECIAL WARNING TO EXPECTANT MOTHERS

Don't Smoke!

Studies have proven both cigarette and marijuana smoking to be damaging to the fetus. According to a study by the National Children's Bureau in Great Britain, babies born to women who smoked during pregnancy had a 30 per cent higher incidence of death at birth than those born to non-smokers. Also, there was a higher frequency of premature births. The American Cancer Society agrees that babies of smoking mothers are generally smaller at birth. Other studies confirm that incidents of premature births are nearly twice as great for smoking mothers than non-smoking mothers and that expectant mothers who smoke have a higher risk of unsuccessful pregnancies resulting from stillbirth and neo-natal death. Newborn babies in a hospital nursery born to mothers who are heavy smokers are nervous and jumpy and do not have the sound sleeping habits possessed by children born to non-smoking mothers. Babies from smoking mothers are easily aroused as noise and other disturbances make them jump and shake, whereas non-smokers' babies sleep the restful, relaxed sleep of a healthy baby.

Nicotine from cigarette smoking also makes it harder for vitamin C in the body to assist in the important function of detoxification, because it is used up in detoxifying the nicotine in the system. Science has observed that non-smoking pregnant women are able to maintain adequate vitamin C levels by taking 35 to 50 milligrams per day while smokers need as high as 300 milligrams to meet the same purpose.

Research on marijuana smoking is proving even more alarming.* Dr. Robert C. Kolodny, head of the Endocrine Research Section at the Masters and Johnson Research Foundation, found that "At least some of the active constituents of marijuana have been shown to cross the placenta." In other words, they reach the fetus. Although he carefully warned that this will have to be confirmed by further research, Dr. Kolodny said: "There may be a significant risk of depressed testosterone levels within the developing fetus when this drug is used by a pregnant woman. Since normal sexual differentiation of the male depends on adequate testosterone stimulation during critical stages of development, it is possible that such development might be disrupted." The question of whether marijuana use can lead to birth of de-

* *Addiction and Drug Abuse Report,* Section One, September 1974, Vol. 5, No. 9.

formed children was answered by Oxford's Professor of Pharmacology, W. D. M. Paton, who flatly warned that those indulging in chronic abuse of the drug ran a serious risk of giving birth to abnormal or defective offspring. He pointed out that administering cannabis at vulnerable periods during pregnancy had been found "to cause fetal death and fetal abnormalities in three species of animals. The deformities include lack of limbs." In these animal experiments, he said, the deformity-producing effect carried over for *two generations* without further exposure to marijuana.

Evidence of "serious damage to cellular processes" was reported by Professor Cecile Leuchtenberger, head of the Department of Cytochemistry at the Swiss Institute for Experimental Cancer Research. She testified: "Smoke of marijuana cigarettes has harmful effects on the tissues and cells of animals and humans. The observations that marijuana cigarette smoke stimulates irregular growth in the respiratory system, that it interferes with DNA stability of cells and chromosomes, that it disturbs the genetic equilibrium, strongly suggest that marijuana cigarette smoke is a health hazard and may," she concludes, "involve the possibilities of lung cancer and genetic damage."

If you smoke and want to quit, now is the perfect time to do so. Many women who were unable to break the habit for themselves, can easily do so for their baby's sake.

Aspirin Can Be Harmful During Pregnancy

According to a study undertaken by Australian physicians, Dr. Edith Collins and Dr. Gillian Turner,† women who take aspirin regularly during pregnancy suffer a high rate of complications including bleeding, infection, and neo-natal death. Aspirin use ranged from two to twelve aspirin doses daily to once a week dosage among the pregnant women tested. Of sixty-three daily aspirin users, four had stillbirths and one baby died after birth. Among eighty-three women who took aspirin less often, but at least once a week, one stillborn and three newborn deaths occurred. Dr. Reba Hill of Baylor University in Houston, Texas, found in her study of 300 pregnant women that 64 per cent of them took analgesic or pain-relieving agents during pregnancy and called the Australian study important "because it shows that anyone taking excessive quantities of aspirin can certainly damage her baby." Based on similar studies, a Food and Drug Administration advisory panel is preparing to recommend that a warning against unprescribed use in pregnancy be placed on every aspirin bottle.

† Published in the British medical journal, *Lancet*, August 23, 1975.

Excessive Use of Alcohol Can Damage Babies

British doctors in the 1800s reported that alcoholism in mothers led to "weak, feeble and distempered children." Modern medicine confirms that alcoholic mothers are far more likely to bear children with birth defects including mental and physical retardation. Dr. David W. Smith, a Seattle, Washington, pediatrician, states that babies born to mothers who are alcoholics look different from ordinary infants because of the alcohol's injurious effect on tissue growth and development with the brain particularly susceptible to damage. Half of the babies born with what Dr. Smith calls fetal alcohol syndrome are mentally deficient when tested two years later. The syndrome afflicts one out of three babies born to mothers who are chronic drinkers. One investigation revealed that of eight children with birth defects, all were born to alcoholic mothers. In another study, only one of nine babies born to mothers who were heavy drinkers was normal. The syndrome does not seem to affect moderate drinkers, although Dr. Smith warns that *any* alcohol a pregnant woman consumes quickly reaches the womb and her unborn baby. The number of babies who are literally "born drunk" is on the rise, and it is imperative that heavy drinkers who want healthy babies give up liquor *before* becoming pregnant.

3

A WORD ABOUT DIET DURING PREGNANCY

The Yogic View

A major source of Prana, or universal energy, is food. Knowing this, the Yogi views diet as playing a major role in accomplishing his goals of regenerating energy and imparting vitality to the body while promoting health, strength, and longevity. What you eat determines how you look, how you feel, and how you function. According to the *Bhagavad Gita,* there are three types of food: *sattvic* food (pure food), *rajasic* food (stimulating food) and *tamasic* food (impure food). Milk, butter, fruits, vegetables, and whole grains come under the category of *sattvic* foods, or those which are good to eat. Spices, meat, fish, and eggs, as well as alcohol, come under the heading of *rajasic* food, or that food which stimulates the nervous system. Food that is impure and not fit to eat comes under the *tamasic* category.

Yogis advocate vegetarianism, believing it to be a healthier way of life. They also object to the killing of innocent animals on ethical and spiritual grounds. However, it is not necessary to become a vegetarian to practice Yoga. Most people continue their established eating habits and derive great benefit through regular practice of Hatha Yogasanas and Pranayama techniques.

The diet of an expectant mother is extremely important as what she eats not only determines her own health, but that of her child as well. A pregnant woman is building in her body the tissues and organs of a new human being. Studies have shown that the rate of development and the viability (ability to live) of the unborn child is largely influenced by the mother's health and nutrition prior to conception and during the first half of pregnancy, and that the size and length of the child at birth is greatly influenced by maternal nutrition during the last half of pregnancy. The developing child has no other source of nutrition but his mother, and poor nutrition may also seriously affect the placental tissues so that the required nutrients may not pass through properly.

Vegetarianism and the Expectant Mother

Proper nutrition is obviously vital during pregnancy. If you are a practicing vegetarian, you will not want to alter your eating habits drastically during pregnancy; however, you will want to be especially careful to maintain a well-balanced diet in order to give your baby the best possible start in life. It is possible for an expectant mother to maintain a vegetarian diet successfully so long as she gets a variety and a balance of necessary proteins, vitamins, and minerals. Vitamins and minerals abound in the vegetable kingdom as well as carbohydrates, fats, and proteins that are in many ways superior to those found in the animal kingdom. By eating a wide variety of foods and by paying particular attention to complementary proteins, a vegetarian mother-to-be may insure an adequate pre-natal diet balanced in the nutrients necessary for the growth and development of a healthy baby.

A vegetarian diet also provides plenty of bulk and roughage which is extemely important and helps to eliminate constipation. Recent studies have shown that a low bulk diet may be associated with increased incidence of cancer of the colon and arteriosclerosis.

If you are not a vegetarian, but are considering becoming one, do wait until after your baby is born before adopting a new dietary system. Animal proteins are the best source of *complete* protein and of a complete balance of amino acids, the necessary building blocks for healthy cell development. Successful vegetarianism calls for a thorough knowledge of nutrition and dietary requirements. Most people, vegetarian and non-vegetarian alike, have a difficult time maintaining a consistently well-balanced daily diet. It is not advisable to eliminate important sources of protein and amino acids at the time when you and your baby need them most.

Life-force Foods

Yogis advocate eating only those foods that impart as much Prana to the body as possible and stress eating a variety of fresh fruits and vegetables, cereals, nuts, and milk and milk products. These foods are called life-force foods and are natural foods—primarily those that grow. They should be eaten as fresh and as close to their natural state as possible and are preferably organically grown. A true Yoga diet avoids all foods that have been processed or denatured by being refined, preserved, canned, pickled, smoked, or "enriched." Chemical additives are unnecessary and may even be harmful, although they are much a part of our present day culture. A yogic diet is centered around *sattvic* or pure foods eaten in an unadulterated state. During pregnancy, you need foods that are rich enough for two in proteins, vitamins, and minerals. Yoga concentrates on the natural foods highest in these values.

Cooking should be minimized in a yogic diet in keeping with the overall aim of eating foods as close to their natural state as possible. High temperatures and long cooking processes alter or destroy important vitamins, minerals, and proteins. Modern dietetic teachings emphasize the necessity of eating raw foods daily. The most revitalizing of all are raw-food meals, so eat as many raw fruits and vegetables as you can. Fresh green salads and fruit salads with homemade dressings make a delicious meal in themselves. During cooking, green vegetables may be steamed just until tender, using a small amount of water, or quickly sautéed oriental style in a little vegetable oil. Not only are they more nutritious prepared in this way, but they are more attractive and taste better too. Root vegetables, such as carrots, potatoes, turnips, and beets, can be baked or steamed in their skins to retain their minerals.

In accordance with Yoga teachings, all strong seasonings, including salt, are to be avoided. Salt is a lifeless food and cutting down on salt retards water retention—a major cause of swelling and bloating during pregnancy—and helps to bypass digestive upsets. Celery or vegetable salt may be substituted instead. Salt is usually not found in fresh fruits and vegetables, but usually is found in large amounts in processed and prepared foods and is another good reason for restricting or avoiding these foods. The average pregnant woman will maintain a normal weight gain of ½ pound a week when she consumes only 25 to 40 salt units and 1,800 calories a day. Some women are particularly sensitive during pregnancy and must eliminate salt from their diets completely.

Protein Without Meat

Protein is the most important food nutrient for pregnant women. The entire body is made up of protein, so all pregnant women need sufficient amounts for themselves and for growth of the fetus and accessory tissues. Yoga students who choose vegetarianism derive quality protein from the following foods:

>   milk and milk products (cottage cheese is good)
>
>   cheese
>
>   yogurt
>
>   nuts
>
>   peanut butter and other nut butters
>
>   seeds (sunflower, sesame, and pumpkin seeds are
>   all good sprinkled on salads or sandwiches)
>
>   legumes (dried peas, beans, and lentils)

avocados

whole grains, cereals and breads

soybeans and soybean products (including tofu and miso)

eggs

Olives and coconuts are also good protein sources if you have a taste for them. Brewer's yeast is a valuable protein supplement if it is fortified; however, read the label as it is 100 per cent carbohydrate if not fortified.

Protein Complementarity

Vegetable proteins contain an excess of some amino acids and a deficiency of others, which make them less usable by the body than animal proteins which contain all the amino acids the body requires. These deficiencies can be matched with amino-acid strengths in other foods, however, to produce protein usability equivalent to meat protein. This effect is called "protein complementarity."*

The combination of milk with cereal or bread in meals where neither meat nor eggs are served is an example of this effect, as the amino-acid strength in milk protein makes those in cereals or bread more useful in the body. In other words, the amino-acid content in both protein forms balance and complement each other. Milk and peanut butter sandwiches form another protein complementarity as the two foods complete each other. Although no new proteins are formed through the combinations of certain specified foods, the body is better able to make use of the amino-acid strengths of each food through the blend. Rice plus beans, wheat plus cheese and breads with added seed meals are further examples of this effect. A festive recipe incorporating the principle of protein complementarity is the traditional Cuban dish, *Arroz Con Frijoles Negros* (Rice with Black Beans).

ARROZ CON FRIJOLES NEGROS

3 cups brown rice, cooked
(1 cup raw rice)

3 cups black beans, cooked
(1½ cup dry black beans)

1 onion, finely chopped

2 cloves garlic, minced

1 green pepper, chopped

1 small (2 oz.) jar pimentos

3 tablespoons olive oil

1 bay leaf

1 teaspoon oregano, crushed

½ lemon

Salt and pepper to taste

* For detailed information on protein complementarity, see Frances Moore Lappe's *Diet for a Small Planet*, Rev. Ed. (New York: Ballantine Books, 1975).

Soak dry beans in water overnight. Add water to make two quarts and cook until tender. Sauté minced garlic, chopped onion and green pepper in olive oil until golden. Add to beans with bay leaf and oregano and simmer 20 minutes. Chop pimentos. Drain beans and reserve liquid to use as a gravy. Lightly toss beans with cooked rice and pimentos. Squeeze lemon juice over all. Add salt and pepper to taste. Reheat to serve. May also be chilled and served as a salad on crisp lettuce leaves with oil and vinegar dressing.

Iron in the Diet

Pregnant women need great quantities of iron as it is transferred to the fetus and placenta in large amounts, especially during the last four months of pregnancy. Blood loss during delivery also requires a back-up supply of iron. Iron builds good blood for you and your baby and aids in the oxidation of food nutrients; lack of iron can lead to miscarriage, fetal malformations, and anemia. It is also necessary to furnish the newborn infant with iron stores he will need for blood formation during the neo-natal period before food sources of iron are added to his diet. Shortly before birth, the infant stores iron and vitamin B_{12} in his system, for these particular nutrients are not readily available to the baby immediately after birth. Therefore, it is most important that the mother have adequate supplies of these nutrients during her pregnancy.

Iron may be found in the following Yoga diet foods:

> dates
> prunes
> raisins
> peaches
> apricots
> cooked dried apricots and other cooked dried fruits
> spinach, beet tops, and other dark-green, leafy vegetables
> wheat germ
> green peas
> dark molasses
> legumes
> nuts

Other good iron sources are eggs, fortified brewer's yeast, whole grain breads and cereals and, if you are not vegetarian, liver and beef. Seaweed and sesame seeds are extremely high in iron content. Iron may also be found in most calcium sources.

Calcium

Why is milk so important in the pre-natal diet? It supplies nearly all the calcium necessary to make good teeth and strong bones for your baby; no other food can take the place of milk or cheese in supplying this mineral. Pregnant women need extra calcium for making the bones of the fetus as calcium is depleted from the skeleton of the mother if there is an inadequate supply during pregnancy. Calcium is also an aid to blood coagulation and muscle contractility for the mother-to-be. Cheese is very high in calcium content while nuts, eggs, and raw, green, leafy vegetables—such as watercress and turnip, daikon, and collard greens—also contain calcium and may act as supplementary foods. Sesame seeds and seaweed are the best sources of all, outside of milk. If pregnant women use these foods, there should be no calcium deficiency unless vitamin D is inadequate.

Vitamin D is important for pregnant women as it promotes absorption and retention of calcium. Good sources include vitamin D milk, butter, egg yolks, fish, and liver. Vitamin D is actually a hormone synthesized in the skin when exposed to the ultra-violet rays of the sun. Exposing the skin to direct sunshine will produce vitamin D. Windows filter out ultra-violet light, so a person has to go outside to absorb the beneficial rays of the sun. Direct sunshine is the best natural source of vitamin D . . . and it's free!

Fluids

Adequate fluids are vital in maintaining the body's metabolism during pregnancy, so remember to drink lots of water. Many expectant mothers cut down on their consumption of coffee and tea or quit drinking them altogether simply because "they don't taste good anymore." Your system is especially sensitive during pregnancy. If you tune into your body, it will tell you what it needs at the time. If you really enjoy coffee or tea, and almost everyone does, it isn't necessary to forego them during your pregnancy, but try to cut down by substituting fresh fruit and vegetable juices, vegetable broths, and herb teas. Herb teas are especially good with a little honey and lemon added to them. Red Raspberry Leaf Tea has long been associated with pregnancy in folklore as an aid to childbirth.

Natural Sweeteners

Do avoid white sugar, which is over-processed and denatured (an "empty food"), and substitute honey or one of the other natural sweeteners instead. Molasses, maple or cane sugar, beet sugar, and fresh or dried fruits are all delicious, satisfying, and nutritious. Pure honey is a perfect sweetening agent. It is rich in vitamins and minerals and is quickly assimilated into the bloodstream. As a food, it is one of the best sources of quick energy. However, if weight gain is a problem, go easy. All sweeteners are a source of unneeded calories.

For an energizing and delicious snack guaranteed to satisfy the sweetest tooth, naturally, try *Arthur Murray's Mix,* a recipe shared by the famous dance master.

ARTHUR MURRAY'S MIX

1 package granola	½ cup wheat germ
1 cup chopped dates	½ cup soy nuts
1 cup chopped apricots (dried)	1 cup grated coconut (optional)
1 cup raisins	
1 cup nuts (walnuts, almonds, pecans, or peanuts)	1 cup pure honey (vary for sweetness desired)
1 cup seeds (sesame seeds are good)	2 to 3 tablespoons dark molasses

Combine all ingredients and spread in shallow pan. Bake in 350° oven for 30 minutes. Stir once and cool in oven. Reheat oven to 200° and bake one hour. Cool in oven and store in covered container.

You Don't Have to Be a Vegetarian!

A primary source of protein in America is meat, especially beef. Many people feel that they just can't give up the meat and meat products they have enjoyed all of their lives. Most doctors feel that it is especially desirable during pregnancy to take a diet containing proteins of animal and vegetable origin in order to insure the proper nutritional balance for both mother and baby, since the price of insufficient protein is permanent damage to the baby.

Including meat in the diet also insures a proper amount of vitamin B_{12}, one of the B complex vitamins important for growth and reproduction, which is the one vitamin not present in sufficient amounts in fresh fruits and vegetables. Most vegetarians develop a deficiency of this vitamin over varying periods of time and must supplement it by taking foods fortified with B_{12}. Miso, a fermented soybean product, is a valuable natural source for B_{12}.

Regular practice of Yoga does not mean that you must automatically become a vegetarian. Yoga means union, harmony, and balance in life. Any diet can be unbalanced, vegetarian or otherwise. A healthy, well-balanced diet that includes plenty of natural foods, raw fruits and vegetables, and a moderate intake of animal foods is well within the goals of Yoga.

Partial Vegetarianism . . . a Post-natal Alternative

As you continue to practice Yoga, you may find that meat does not appeal to you and you may discover yourself craving the lighter, more natural foods instead. This does not mean that you must become an instant vegetarian! A satisfying alternative to the vegetarian question for many, after the baby arrives, is partial vegetarianism. In these days of inflation and skyrocketing food prices, it makes sense to cut down on meat consumption. You may decide to serve meat, fish, or chicken once or twice a week and find it surprisingly sufficient, discovering that with a little planning, your body and your budget will both benefit.

Fasting

Pregnancy is definitely not the time to fast. An expectant mother needs all of the nutrients she can get for the body-building process that is taking place within. The baby will take what he needs from his mother's system, so the pregnant woman needs enough vitamins, minerals, and proteins to cover the baby's development and to maintain her own bodily processes as well. The baby's cells and organs are being formed every day, so good daily nutrition is vital to the health of those cells and organs. It is not healthy for you or your baby to go without good food for even a day during pregnancy. Fasting can be a healthful, cleansing experience, but *not* during pregnancy.

CHAPTER

4

PRANAYAMA TECHNIQUES . . . AS NATURAL AS BREATHING

What Is Pranayama?

Prana means universal energy. Yogis believe that the entire universe is permeated with this vital energy. Although Prana is found in all the elements, most of the Prana we extract for our bodies is in the air that we breathe, and it is possible through conscious breathing techniques to store up this energy in the body. By deliberately concentrating and controlling our breath with awareness, we are able to energize and revitalize our body. The knowledge and control of Prana through breathing is called Pranayama or Yogic Breathing.

Breathing is the most vital of the bodily functions, the very essence of life. Each cell in the body is sustained by oxygen, and a sufficient amount of oxygen is a must for a healthy body. Most of the time we breathe unconsciously with shallow breathing using only about one third of our lung capacity. Yogic Breathing is deep breathing, with awareness, which concentrates on expanding the lungs to their full capacity. By becoming aware of our breathing and by practicing certain simple breathing techniques, it is possible to expand the lung capacity, thereby increasing oxygen intake and greatly energizing the body.

Benefits of Deep Breathing

During pregnancy, there is an even greater need for proper oxygen metabolism as the body is not only maintaining and replenishing cell life, but constructing the cells of a new being. Brain cells are particularly demanding of sufficient oxygen for proper functioning as the brain requires three times the amount of oxygen used by all of the rest of the body.

25

Deep breathing, using the full lung capacity, provides oxygen for the entire system and offsets tension and that all too familiar "tired feeling." Through Pranayama techniques, the body is relaxed and energized at the same time. With regular practice of Yogic Deep Breathing, digestion is improved, health and vitality are increased, and a feeling of well-being is experienced.

It is a good practice to perform a few deep-breathing exercises upon arising and before going to bed at night. Always practice breathing exercises in a well-ventilated room or out of doors. Deep breathing should always be performed in a relaxed state without raising the shoulders or chest during respiration.

Abdominal Breathing

The purpose of breathing exercises is to direct Prana to the solar plexus, a seat of vital energy, and to other parts of the body with recharging and revitalizing effects. Yogic Breathing is abdominal breathing as opposed to upper chest breathing and concentrates on the use of the abdomen during Pranayama techniques. Only by utilizing the abdomen during the breathing process is it possible to inhale fully and completely, filling the lungs with life-giving oxygen.

Yogic Breathing is rhythmic breathing with inhalation and exhalation receiving the same count. In abdominal breathing, the abdomen expands during inhalation and contracts during exhalation. As the diaphragm descends, the abdomen expands while the chest is also expanded by elevation of the ribs. This causes the lungs to be filled with air. This is all done in one movement, smoothly and without jerking or separation. During exhalation the diaphram is lifted, drawing in the stomach, and the ribs return to normal position as the air is expelled from the lungs.

Nasopharyngeal Breathing

Nasopharyngeal Breathing is a form of deep breathing that may be done at any time, in any place, and in almost any position. It is a simple but effective method of abdominal breathing whereby concentration is centered on the nasopharyngeal passage. The air is inhaled through the nostrils during this technique, and the breath is drawn into the nasopharynx with the nostrils remaining passive. The same is true during exhalation, although a slight effort is made to contract the throat—but not the nostrils—and a faint sound

kept closed during the entire respiration cycle. The
ring inhalation and contract during exhalation. Re-
when doing Nasopharyngeal Breathing and do not
breath. The following technique for Nasopharyngeal
an exercise and should be treated as such; do not attempt to
athe this way all of the time.

NASOPHARYNGEAL BREATHING

TECHNIQUE:

1. Settle into a comfortable position. Slowly inhale with the mouth closed,
   drawing the air in through the pharyngeal passage behind the throat.
   Nostrils remain stationary throughout. Allow the air to fill the lower part
   of the lungs, then the middle, then the upper. The abdomen will expand
   during inhalation. Inhale to count of 4.

2. Exhale *slowly* to count of 4, compressing the air through your throat and
   slowly contracting the ribs and abdomen. Continue in this manner for 6
   breaths. Rest. Remember not to raise your chest or shoulders as this
   results in upper-chest breathing.

BENEFITS: Nasopharyngeal Breathing is a basic form of deep breathing conducive to relaxation, easing tension of both body and mind. Useful during the
early stages of labor to combat the muscular tension that produces pain.

Breathing Techniques for Quick Energy

The Deep-breathing Asana, the Ha Breath or Cleansing Breath and Kapalbhati or Recharging Breath are recommended as energizing techniques
and may be practiced at any time during pregnancy when fatigue is felt.
Remember not to strain while performing these techniques as they are most
beneficial when performed in a relaxed manner.

During practice of these techniques, the system is flooded with oxygen and
Prana and revitalized in a completely natural and healthful way. If at any
time dizziness or light-headedness occurs or vision is impaired, immediately
stop the exercise and lie down in Savasana until the feeling passes. It is possible to hyperventilate while doing deep-breathing exercises if the system is
unused to Pranayama techniques. Breathing into a paper bag helps to restore
the carbon dioxide level to its proper balance.

DEEP-BREATHING ASANA

1. Stand with feet together and spine erect. Clasp hands under the chin with fingers interlocked and palms together.

2. Inhale deeply through the nostrils with mouth closed and head stationary, raising elbows toward the ceiling. Fingers remain locked while palms separate. Hands touch chin at all times.

3. Exhale completely through the throat passage with mouth open, bringing elbows together as you push your head back.

4. Inhale and bring head slowly down to starting position, again raising elbows. (By raising your arms to the sides, you automatically expand the rib cage allowing lungs to fill completely with air.)

5. Repeat for 10 breaths. Eyes remain open throughout or dizziness may occur. Rest with arms relaxed at sides for 20 seconds. Repeat a second set.

BENEFITS: This Asana should always be done before beginning any exercise session as it awakens the body by increasing the general circulation and flooding the lungs with life-giving oxygen.

HA BREATH (Cleansing Breath)

TECHNIQUE:

1. Stand with legs apart. Inhale deeply through the nostrils, raising the arms sidewise until they are stretched above the head.

2. Bend forward from the waist, at the same time expelling the breath through the mouth making the sound, "HA." Relax the body and let the arms and head hang loosely as you repeat the "HA" sound several times.

3. Stand up slowly and repeat twice.

BENEFITS: The Ha or Cleansing Breath completely fills the lungs with fresh air and expels all stale air that is lying in them. It refreshens and recharges the body at any time when fatigue is felt.

KAPALBHATI (Blowing or Recharging Breath)

TECHNIQUE:

1. Sit in Vajrasana (Fixed Firm Pose) with hands on the knees. Concentrate on one spot in the distance.

2. Blow out through pursed lips, expelling the breath by *gently* contracting the abdomen in a rhythmic manner, giving each breath one count. Spine should be straight.

3. Practice from 10 to 25 counts, gradually increasing the number.

BENEFITS: This is an energizing or a recharging technique. It may be practiced during pregnancy whenever you feel the need for a "boost" of energy, and it is a good way to end your Yoga practice before resting in Savasana. This is the breathing done during transition and the final stages of labor when the contractions have begun to accelerate and intensify. The rhythm of Kapalbhati may be speeded up as the contractions become harder. Special care must be taken not to hyperventilate while performing this breathing technique.

Breathing Techniques to Relax By

The Complete Breath, Alternate-Nostril Breathing, and *Sitale Breathing* are recommended as relaxation techniques. Tension is eased through practice of these exercises and replaced by a calm and serene frame of mind. These Pranayama techniques are natural tranquilizers and may be practiced daily during pregnancy.

THE COMPLETE BREATH

TECHNIQUE:

1. Exhale deeply. Inhale through the nostrils as slowly and as smoothly as you can. Gently extend the abdomen by pushing out with the abdominal muscles as you inhale. Completely fill the lungs and expand the chest as much as possible.

2. Without pausing, slowly exhale through the nostrils so that the body returns to its beginning position. Again, without pause, slowly inhale, concentrating on the breath with awareness of the energy within you as you perform this technique.

BENEFITS: The Complete Breath relieves tension and promotes calm. This is excellent preparation for childbirth and will help during the first stage of labor, which is the longest, to relax between and during contractions.

NOTE: The Complete Breath may be practiced lying down or in a standing or sitting position.

ALTERNATE-NOSTRIL BREATHING (Moon-Sun Breath)

TECHNIQUE:

1. Close your eyes and lightly place the index and middle fingers on the forehead with the tip of your thumb on your right nostril and your other fingers on the left.

2. Close your right nostril by pressing the thumb against it and inhale a slow, complete breath through your left nostril to a silent count of 6.

3. Keep your thumb pressed on the right nostril and close the left with your ring and little fingers. Hold the breath for the count of 6.

4. Remove the thumb from the right nostril and keep the left closed. Exhale slowly through the right nostril to the count of 6.

5. Without pausing, repeat the entire process in reverse. Close left nostril, inhale through right; close both, hold; release left nostril and exhale. This completes one round. Do 6 rounds with a steady count of 6 beats.

BENEFITS: This is an excellent natural tranquilizer and promotes calm and relaxation.

SITALE BREATHING

TECHNIQUE:

1. Sitale Breathing may be done in Vajrasana (Fixed Firm Pose), Sukhasana (Easy Pose) or Savasana. Assume the posture and concentrate on one spot in the distance or on the floor about 4 feet in front of you.

2. Inhale slowly through the mouth concentrating on the throat passage called the oropharynx. This is the air passage between the mouth and the larynx. Just as a valve regulates the air in a radiator, so the larynx regulates the breath of the body. Draw the air in slowly, making a noise "AH," to the count of 8. (Count may be adjusted for individual comfort; the important point to remember is that the inhalation and exhalation be of the same duration.)

3. When the point of maximum inhalation is reached, exhale, closing the larynx to make the sound "KEE," to the count of 8. Repeat 6 times. This technique will improve with practice.

BENEFITS: This completely natural breathing technique has a tranquilizing effect, taking the mind away from the body and easing the tension which causes pain. As one concentrates on this Pranayama technique, awareness of external factors gradually fades. Sitale breathing is actually a Pranayama technique for meditation. In India, one advanced yogi adept in Pranayama was observed to alleviate his heart attack by using Sitale Breathing. This is an extremely effective method to utilize during the early stages of labor.

Yogic Breathing and Techniques
Taught in Prepared-childbirth Classes

Pregnant women in prepared-childbirth classes are taught types of breathing exercises based on Yogic Breathing or Pranayama techniques. Concentration on certain of these techniques during labor diminishes pain and allows the mother control by which to assist naturally in the birth of her baby in full consciousness of the birth process. Through concentration on the prepared-breathing techniques rehearsed before labor begins, the mind is unable to concentrate on the "pain" of the uterine contractions. Through actual performance of the breathing techniques, labor can be speeded up and made easier for both mother and baby. Proper breathing assures adequate oxygenation of the blood and supplies the working muscles, including the uterus, with oxygen needed for maximum efficiency during the birth process. Controlled relaxation is also made possible, thereby easing the tension which causes pain.

These breathing exercises, which permit mothers to take an active part during their labors with the ability to guide and control its progress, are vital to prepared-childbirth methods as each breath has its effect toward the goal of a smooth, efficient labor and an unobstructed and joyous birth.

Although psychoprophylactic techniques related to childbirth are based on Pranayama breathing methods, there are certain modifications of the techniques as taught in prepared-childbirth classes. Slow, deliberate chest breathing is sometimes taught as opposed to abdominal breathing during the early stages of labor so as not to interfere with the uterine contractions. However, full abdominal breathing, which lowers the diaphragm and helps the uterus to expel the baby during delivery, is taught for use during the actual birth process.

Childbirth is hard work. The body has an increased need for oxygen when very active and a decreased need when at rest. This principle is observed during the succeeding stages of labor and the breathing techniques are designed accordingly. A deep cleansing breath is always taken before and immediately after each breathing technique. This is a full sighing breath, similar to the Ha Breath, in that air is inhaled through the nostrils and expelled through the mouth. This is the start and the stop of each exercise.

The first breathing technique is used during the early stages of labor when contractions are fairly light. Concentration is centered on one point on the wall or ceiling. (Some women find it helpful to include a special poster for this purpose when packing their hospital bag.) A rhythmic breathing of from 6 to 9 counts with inhalation through the nose and exhalation through the mouth is taught. This is a form of Sitale Breathing, although a slow chest breathing may be taught. The Complete Breath may also be utilized during the first stage of labor and is different only in that it gently involves the abdomen.

The second technique, called accelerated-decelerated shallow breathing, is the panting breath and starts with a steady 4/4 beat accelerating and decelerating with the force of the contraction. Breathe in and out through the mouth with a shallow breath barely reaching the back of the throat. Increase the breathing as the contraction builds to a rapid rhythm and decrease as the contraction slows down. As the contraction builds in strength, the uterine muscles need more oxygen to work with, so you must breathe faster. This panting breath is a light and accelerated form of Kapalbhati with the mouth open.

The third technique is several short, shallow breaths with a short blowing-out breath. To practice, take from 2 to 6 superficial breaths and then exhale with a blowing breath through pursed lips. This technique is helpful during transition, the last stage of labor preceding delivery. This technique also thwarts the urge to push prematurely. If the contractions and the urge to bear down become overwhelmingly strong, Kapalbhati or Blowing is used and is the *only* method that will suffice at this time.

When the time to push comes, take two complete abdominal breaths and hold the third, filling the lungs completely and bringing them to bear directly on the uterus through the diaphragm and the abdominal muscles. At the same time, relax the pelvic floor muscles and *push*, exhale completely, inhale, and push again, usually three times during one contraction. After each series of pushes, be sure to take several deep breaths to maintain an adequate blood-oxygen level.

These are the basic breathing techniques taught in most prepared-childbirth classes. If you are attending such a class, you may find slight variations in method, and you would want to adhere to that teaching. However, all breathing techniques taught in prepared-childbirth classes have their roots in Pranayama.

CHAPTER
5

ANTE-NATAL ASANAS

SUGGESTED PRACTICE SCHEDULE
OF ANTE-NATAL ASANAS

Hold each posture 10 seconds unless otherwise specified; two sets each pose. When a variation is given, do one set each.

SAVASANA

Savasana is the Number One Yoga posture. Sometimes called the Dead Man's Pose or the Sponge, it can be mastered by anyone the first time around and is an excellent posture for relaxation. Daily practice of Savasana during pregnancy is essential and so pleasant that it easily becomes a habit.

Savasana must be practiced in conjunction with the other Asanas. The relaxation following a posture is in actuality a part of that posture and must always be included in your practice of Yoga. Unless the tension of holding a posture is followed by complete relaxation, or release of that tension, the benefits of the posture are negated. When you are in an Asana, certain parts of your body are tightly compressed for 10 or 20 seconds and the veins and arteries in these areas are "dammed up," so to speak, considerably slowing the circulation of the bloodstream. When the posture is relaxed, there is a surge in the blood flow, circulation is enhanced, and the entire body is toned up. This explains why you sometimes feel a pleasurable sensation of warmth in certain areas of your body following an Asana. By practicing Savasana after a posture, the blood is allowed to return to it's normal flow and the tensed muscles are made soft and pliable. Usually, the duration of relaxation in Savasana is the same as for the Asana itself, unless specifically mentioned otherwise.

To assume Savasana, simply lie down on the floor flat on your back with your arms at your sides, palms facing upward. Close your eyes, take several deep breaths and relax. Start with the tips of your toes, concentrate on relaxing them completely and feel all tension drain out of them. Then relax your feet by focusing your full concentration on your feet alone. In the same way, concentrate on relaxing your legs, thighs, trunk, back, etc. by gradually letting go of that part of your body. (Guard against contracting any part of your body already relaxed, when trying to relax another part.) Continue to relax your shoulders, arms, hands, and fingertips. Concentrate on letting go of your scalp, forehead, eyelids, jaws, and chin. You will be amazed at how much tension you will find in these areas. Now feel how heavy your body seems to be. Feel yourself gradually melting into the floor and feel that you are becoming a part of that floor. Lie quietly and enjoy the marvelous sense of well-being that comes with total relaxation.

Now try to visualize a peaceful scene or a favorite place of relaxation. If you imagine you are at the seashore, actually smell the salt air and feel the ocean breezes against your skin as you wiggle your toes in the warm sand and listen to the sea gulls cry. Really *be* there through the power of your imagination. Or you may empty your mind of all thought and make it completely blank. This is harder to achieve and takes some practice. Either way, remember to relax your mind along with your body. Peace of mind is a natural and essential part of full relaxation.

During pregnancy, full support must be provided for all parts of the body so that no muscle is tensed or drawn taut in order for full relaxation to occur. For this reason, it may be desirable to use a rolled towel or pillow under the head or neck (but not the shoulders) and under each knee to increase comfort during Savasana. This will relieve any strain on muscles in the back of the neck and calves.

If tension is felt in the lower back as pregnancy advances from the pressure of the baby's weight upon the spine, this discomfort may be alleviated by bending the knees, elevating the legs, and propping pillows under the calf muscles. Savasana may then be practiced in this position with full benefits of relaxation.

A variation of this posture is to bend the knees to the most comfortable angle, feet flat on the floor. The middle of the back should sink into the floor and there should be no strain at all around the stomach or under the ribs.

Savasana should be practiced throughout pregnancy at any time during the day when fatigue is felt. Set aside a daily rest time, apart from your Yoga practice, in which to relax completely in Savasana. Both you and your baby will benefit.

TECHNIQUES, VARIATIONS, AND BENEFITS
FOR STANDING, PRONE, CROSS-LEGGED,
AND SITTING POSTURES

DEEP-BREATHING ASANA

TECHNIQUE:

1. Stand with feet together and spine erect. Clasp hands under the chin with fingers interlocked and palms together.

2. Inhale deeply through the nostrils with mouth closed while raising elbows toward the ceiling. Fingers remain locked while palms separate. Hands touch chin at all times.

3. Exhale through the throat passage with mouth open, bringing elbows together as you push your head back.

4. Inhale while bringing head slowly down to starting position, again raising elbows. (By raising your arms to the sides, you automatically expand the rib cage, allowing the lungs to fill completely with air.)

5. Repeat for 10 breaths. Eyes remain open throughout or dizziness may occur.

6. Rest with arms relaxed at sides for 20 seconds. Repeat a second set.

BENEFITS: This Asana should always be done before beginning any exercise session as it awakens the body by increasing the general circulation and flooding the lungs with life-giving oxygen.

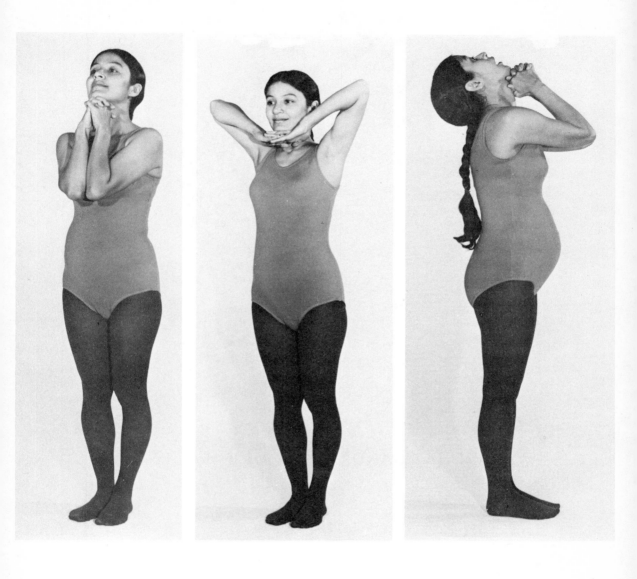

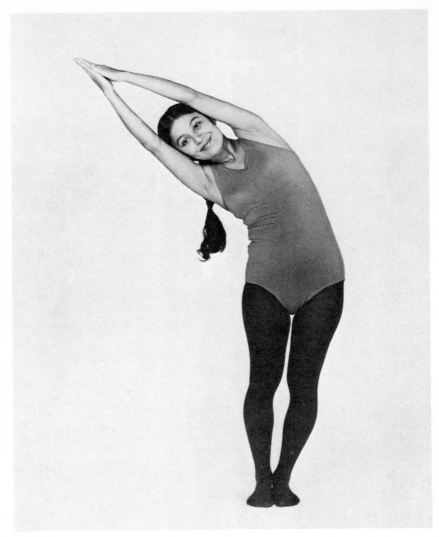

ARDHA-CHANDRASANA (Half Moon Pose)

TECHNIQUE:

1. Stand erect with feet together.

2. Slowly raise arms sidewise above head until palms are together with thumbs crossed in Namascar* position, elbows straight.

3. Gently stretch arms up toward the ceiling and bend slowly to the right as far as possible without twisting the body. Arms and head should move as one unit.

* Namascar is the traditional hand position employed during the Indian greeting or salutation, with palms together, fingers extended together, and thumbs crossed one upon the other.

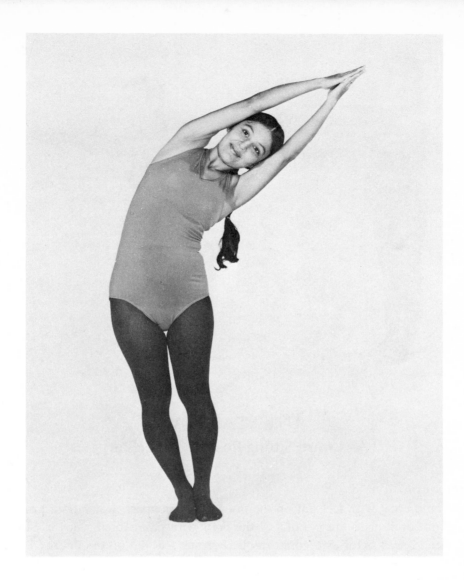

4. Hold for count of 10.

5. Slowly straighten position. Again stretch up and bend to the left without twisting the body.

6. Hold for count of 10.

7. Slowly straighten position and lower arms to the sides with palms down.

8. Rest in position 20 seconds. Repeat a second set. Rest.

BENEFITS: Strengthens the abdominal wall. Improves the sidewise movements of the spine to make it more flexible.

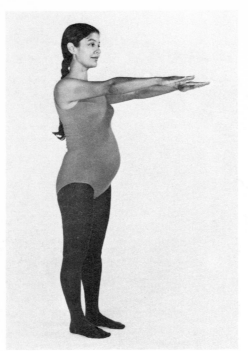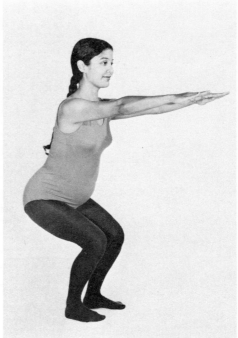

UTKATASANA
(Awkward Sitting Pose)   Three Parts

TECHNIQUE:

1. Stand erect with feet flat on the floor 6 inches apart. Raise both arms in front until arms are parallel to the floor with palms facing down. Slowly bend knees as far as is comfortable, keeping feet flat on the floor. (Try to imagine yourself sitting in a straight-backed chair.) Hold position, arms extended, for 10 seconds. Slowly straighten to standing position.

2. Keeping arms extended, raise up on the toes and slowly bend knees to sitting position while maintaining your balance. Hold 10 seconds, rise up and relax feet in standing position flat on the floor.

3. Again raise up on the toes and slowly bend knees, with both knees touching, until you are sitting on your heels. Hold 10 seconds. Slowly straighten to standing position with feet flat and lower arms to the sides. Relax in standing posture. Repeat.

BENEFITS: This Asana is especially helpful during pregnancy as it strengthens the childbearing muscles by limbering up the pelvic joints, stretching the adductor or riding muscles of the inner thigh and exercising the perineal floor and hip joints. It increases circulation and helps develop balance (an aid in your changing posture during pregnancy).

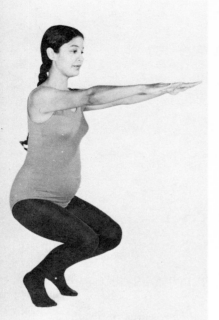
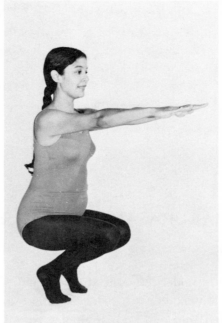
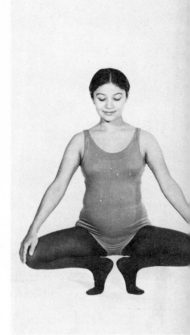

VARIATION FOR UTKATASANA
(Awkward Sitting Pose)

TECHNIQUE:

1. Same as for Utkatasana up to third part.
2. Rise up on toes with knees touching and slowly bend knees until you are sitting on your heels.
3. Place hands on knees and stretch legs wide apart while keeping spine straight. Be careful to keep your balance so you won't tumble over. Hold 10 seconds.
4. Bring knees together and slowly rise to standing position. Lower feet to floor and rest 10 seconds. Repeat. This is an especially good exercise to prepare the childbearing muscles for delivery.

GARURASANA (The Eagle Pose)

TECHNIQUE:

1. Wrap right arm under left arm at elbow and place palms together with thumbs crossed in Namascar.

2. Balance on left foot and wrap right leg over left leg crossing at thigh. Bend knees to accommodate posture and hook right foot behind left calf.

3. Straighten spine while maintaining balance, tighten posture and hold for 10 seconds.

4. Unwind and change sides.

5. Wrap left arm under right arm. Balance on right foot and wrap left leg over right, hooking left foot around right calf. Tighten and hold 10 seconds.

6. Unwind and rest 20 seconds in standing position. Repeat.

BENEFITS: Tones up leg and thigh muscles while developing balance and nerve co-ordination.

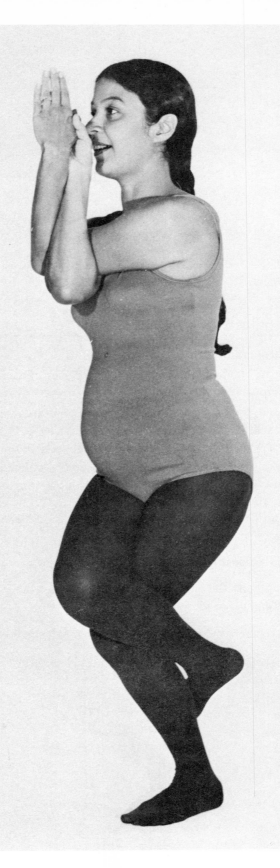

DANDAYAMANA-DHANURASANA
(Standing Bow Pose)

TECHNIQUE:

1. Balance on left leg with left knee locked.

2. Catch inside right ankle with right hand in a firm grip with thumb and fingers together, thumb toward ceiling.

3. Stretch left arm out in front of body with fingers extended in a straight line pointing upward at a 45° angle.

4. Gradually bend forward with left arm extended in front of body and slowly kick back and up with the right foot. Be careful *not to strain* but enjoy the marvelous stretch. Hold for 10 seconds maintaining balance. (This may take some practice. If you do lose your balance, relax the posture and begin again. Never try to recover your balance while maintaining a position.)

5. Rest in standing position for 20 seconds. Change sides. Hold left leg while balancing on right leg and kick back and up. Hold 10 seconds.

6. Relax in standing position.

BENEFITS: Strengthens the muscles in the lower back and helps to relieve the backache so common in pregnancy.

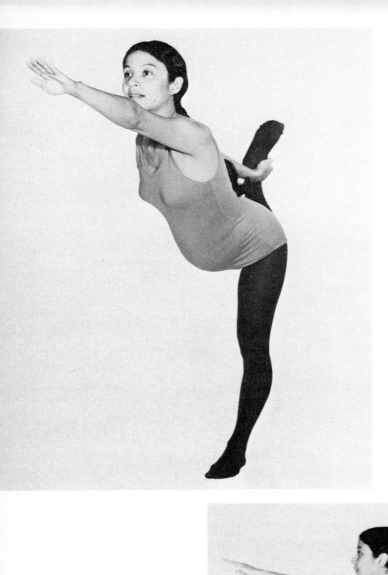

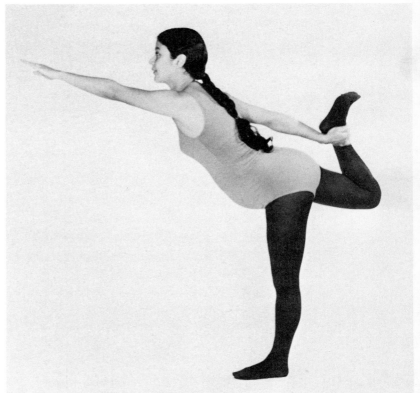

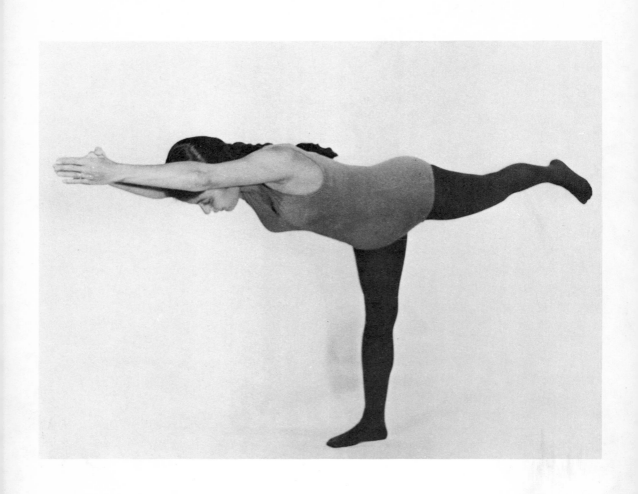

TULADANDASANA (Balancing Stick Pose)

TECHNIQUE:

1. Stand straight with feet together. Raise arms from sides over the head bringing palms together in Namascar, elbows straight.

2. Step forward two feet with right foot. Shift weight forward by bending at the waist and lower body with arms and head together as one unit. At the same time, lift the left leg, with knee locked, to the rear. (It is very important in all standing postures that the knee of the leg on which you are standing remains locked. This stabilizes the posture and helps maintain balance.)

3. The body should now be as straight as a stick (hence the name of the pose) and in one line parallel to the floor. Have another person check to see how straight you are as it's very difficult to judge yourself when in the posture.

4. Hold the pose, with normal breathing, for 10 seconds or as long as is comfortable for you to do so *without straining*.

5. Slowly step back to upright position, arms still extended above head. Change feet and step out two feet in front with the left leg and repeat pose. Hold 10 seconds.

6. Return to upright position slowly and with control. Lower arms to sides, palms down, and relax.

7. A second set of this Asana may be done, but often one set of Tuladandasana is sufficient during pregnancy. Your body will tell you what is right for you.

BENEFITS: This posture affords relief from the pressure of the baby's weight upon your pelvis and lower abdomen during the latter half of pregnancy. It also strengthens calf and thigh muscles and promotes circulation.

TADASANA (Tree Pose)

TECHNIQUE:

1. In standing position, balance on left leg with left knee locked. Slowly raise right leg with foot in front of left leg. (Use your left hand to help raise foot.) Fix right foot into place as close to the groin as possible. Right knee should point down toward the floor. *Do not strain.* This should be a comfortable position. Your foot may come to rest anywhere between the knee and groin.

2. Spine remains straight. Eyes look straight ahead at one point on the wall or on a point on the floor about 4 feet in front of the body.

3. If your foot remains in position without slipping, gradually remove hands and place in Namascar position in front of chest. Shoulders and elbows should be relaxed.

4. Hold posture for 10 seconds. Change sides.

5. Balance on right foot and bring left leg up. Hold 10 seconds.

6. Relax for 20 seconds and repeat pose. Once mastered, this posture has a very serene and soothing effect.

BENEFITS: Helps to improve posture and balance. Exercises the knee joints and stimulates joint secretions eliminating stiffness and enhancing circulation in lower limbs. Increases general circulation and oxygen intake and aids in relaxation.

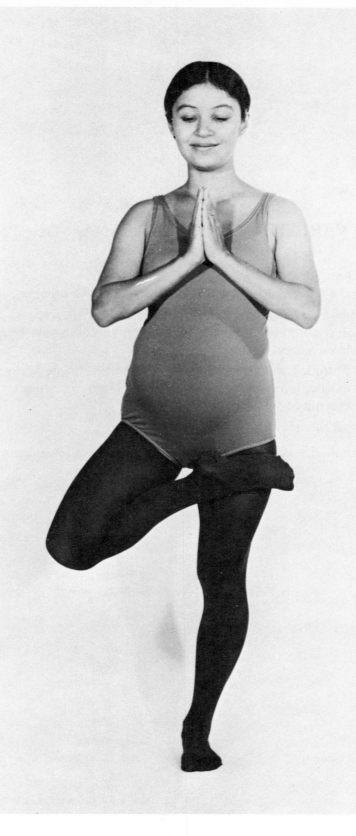

VARIATION FOR TADASANA (Tree Pose)

TECHNIQUE:

1. Stand with both feet together and spine erect. Concentrate vision on one spot on the floor 4 feet in front of you.

2. Inhale to count of 5 as you raise arms to the sides above head with palms coming together.

3. Hold position and slowly exhale to count of 5. Inhale again to count of 5 and exhale. Inhale once more and slowly lower arms to sides while exhaling to count of 5.

4. Repeat 6 times and rest in standing position.

This Variation may be more comfortable to perform toward the end of pregnancy.

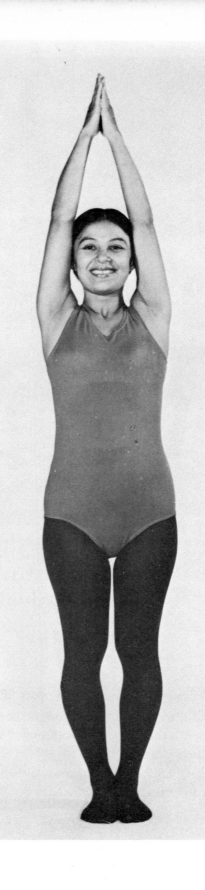

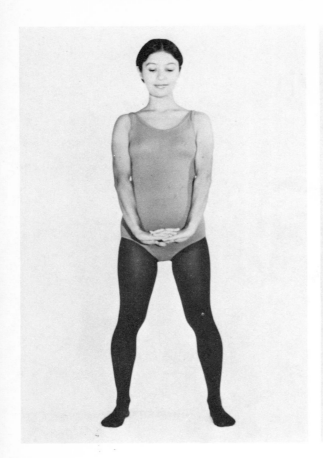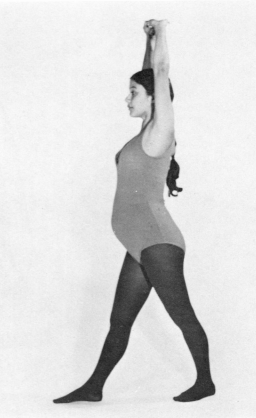

DANDAYAMANA-BIBHAKTAPADASANA
(Standing Separate Leg Pose)

TECHNIQUE:

1. Stand with feet approximately 3 feet apart facing front.

2. Pivot body to the right by turning on the heels until the right foot is in a straight line with the body. Left foot may flair out slightly to keep body balanced. Knees are straight.

3. Inhale to count of 5 and raise arms with fingers interlaced and palms facing away from body to avoid head.

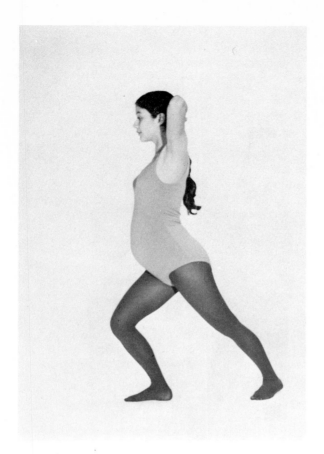

4. Exhale to count of 5 and slowly lunge forward dropping hands to back of neck. Spine remains straight with main weight of body centered in lower hips.

5. Inhale to count of 5 and slowly straighten position raising arms above head.

6. Exhale to count of 5, lunge forward again, and repeat position.

7. Repeat 4 times on right side.

8. Return to front-facing position, lower hands, and rest 20 seconds.

9. Repeat entire procedure on left side 4 times.

10. Return to front-facing position, lower arms to sides, and rest.

BENEFITS: Strengthens lower spine, calf muscles, and upper thighs. Aids in improving posture and breath control.

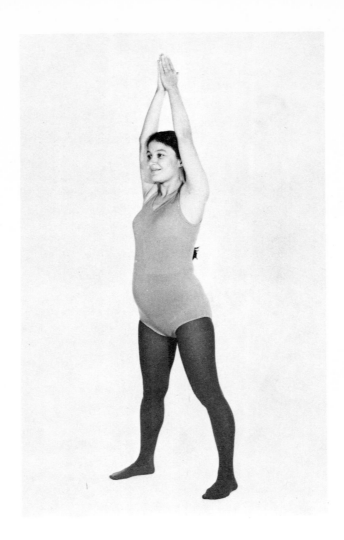

PRASARITA PADOTTANASANA
(Standing Separate Leg Stretching Pose)

TECHNIQUE:

1. Face front in standing position with knees straight. Spread legs apart to a comfortable distance (3 or 4 feet) keeping feet parallel.

2. Slowly raise arms to the sides while inhaling to count of 5 until palms are together.

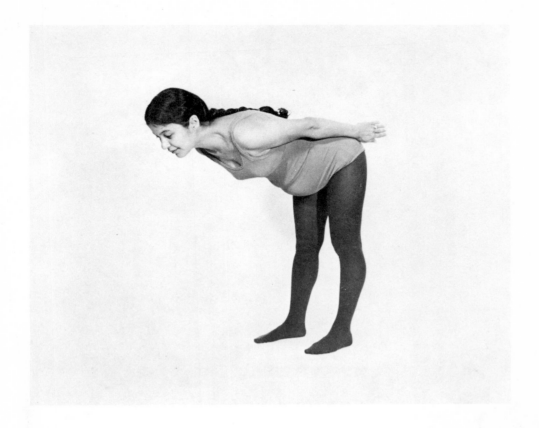

3. Slowly bend forward, exhaling to count of 5 while lowering arms to the side keeping them in line with the sides of the body.

4. Bend forward to waist length. Upper torso should be parallel to the floor at point of maximum exhalation.

5. Inhale to count of 5 and slowly return to upright position, raising arms in line with sides of the body to above head.

6. Repeat 6 times. On last exhalation, remain in upright position and slowly lower arms to sides. Rest in standing position.

BENEFITS: Exercises lower back and relieves abdominal pressure. Helps develop powers of concentration and breath control.

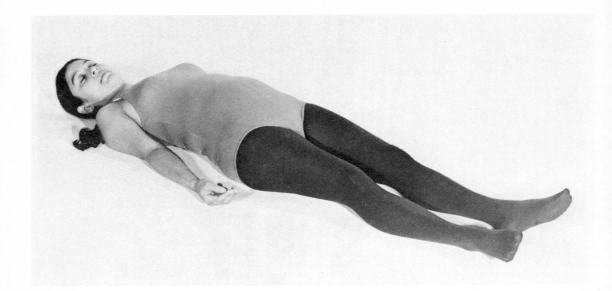

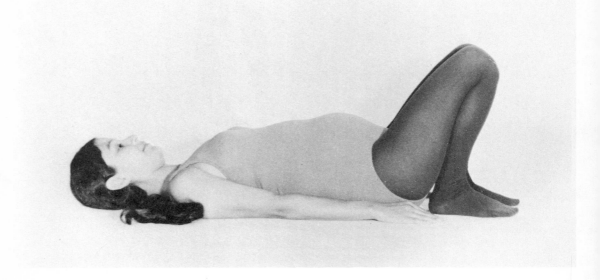

DEVIPADAPEETHAM (The Bridge)

TECHNIQUE:

1. Lie on your back in Savasana with eyes closed.
2. Draw legs up with knees bent as close to the buttocks as is comfortable. Feet are flat on the floor about 6 inches apart. Arms should be straight at your sides with palms down.

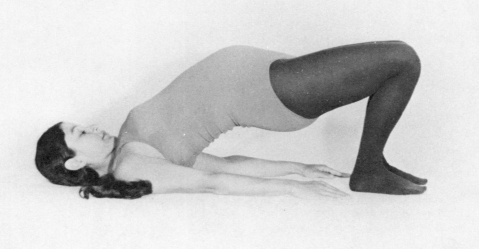

3. Slowly lift the bottom part of your spine off the floor, shifting your weight toward your knees and heels.

4. Inhale slowly to count of 5 while arching your back into a bridge. Arms remain stationary on floor.

5. Without pausing and retaining the breath, slowly exhale to count of 5, and lower back to supine position with bottom of the spine leading the movement.

6. Repeat for 4 cycles. Rest in Savasana.

VARIATION FOR DEVIPADAPEETHAM

TECHNIQUE:

1. Follow steps 1 through 4.

2. While in the bridge position, inhale and exhale one full breath to count of 5. Inhale again and slowly lower the body as you exhale to count of 5.

3. Repeat for 4 cycles including the extra breath each time you hold the bridge position.

BENEFITS: This exercise is especially effective in relieving the lower back-ache often experienced by pregnant women.

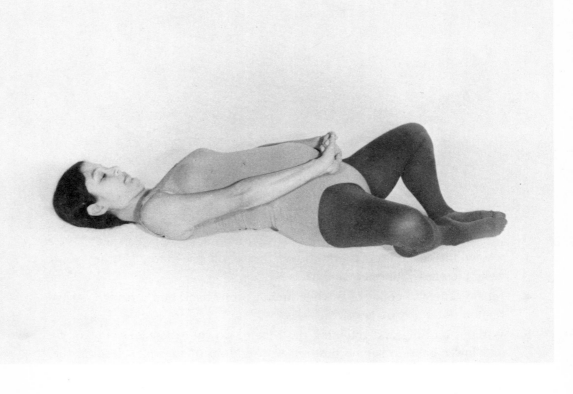

SUPTA-KONASANA (Thigh Stretch)

TECHNIQUE:
1. Lie on your back in Savasana with eyes closed and chin tucked down into notch between collarbone.
2. Draw legs up, soles of feet touching, allowing bent knees to open outward and fall as close to the floor as possible without straining.
3. Interlock fingers of both hands and turn palms out from body, resting hands on pelvic bone.

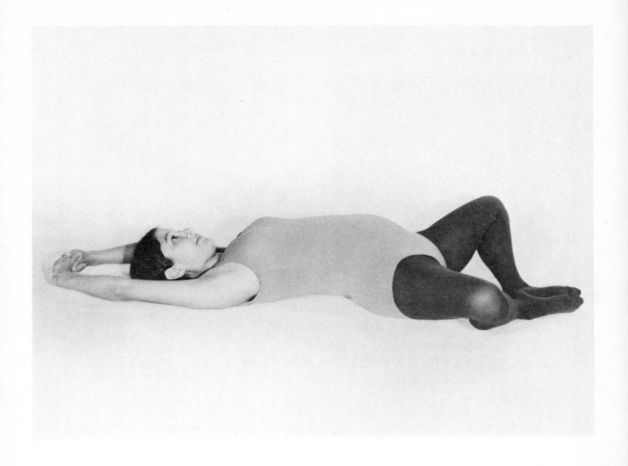

4. Inhale to count of 5 and raise arms above head until hands touch the floor. Try to keep elbows straight.

5. Without pausing and retaining the breath, exhale slowly to count of 5 and return arms to original position.

6. Repeat 6 times. Rest in Savasana.

BENEFITS: This Asana is important to practice during the last two months of pregnancy as it strengthens the pelvic floor muscles used in giving birth by stretching pelvic joints, perineal, and inner thigh muscles. This is a good position in which to lie while resting during the latter part of pregnancy and is also an excellent position in which to practice diaphragmatic breathing or panting breath used during delivery.

ANTE-NATAL ASANAS   61

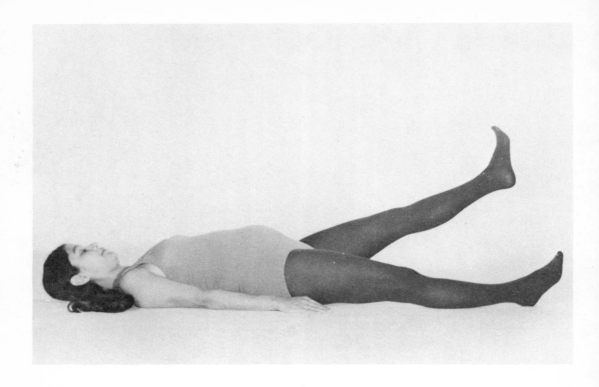

UTTHITA-PADASANA (Leg Lifting Pose)

TECHNIQUE:

1. Lie down in Savasana. Tilt pelvis, pressing small of back firmly against floor, and hold throughout exercise.

2. Breathe in slowly to count of 5 as you raise right leg with right ankle bent to 90° angle. (Do not point the toe in this posture. By bending your ankle, you escape the leg cramps which often occur during pregnancy.) Keep right knee straight and left knee perfectly flat.

3. Breathe out to count of 5 as you slowly lower leg and raise head. (Don't forget to maintain pelvic tilt.)

4. Repeat left side. Lower leg and rest 10 seconds.

5. Raise both legs together, knees locked, 2 inches from floor and hold 10 seconds. Slowly lower legs to floor and rest in Savasana.

BENEFITS: Strengthens abdominal muscles and aids in the removal of gas from intestines. Helps offset added pressure on pelvic joints from the expanding uterus during pregnancy, which affects blood vessels and can lead to leg cramps and varicose veins. Promotes limberness and muscle tone in pelvic region and helps increase elasticity of the pelvic floor. Releases tension and aids during delivery.

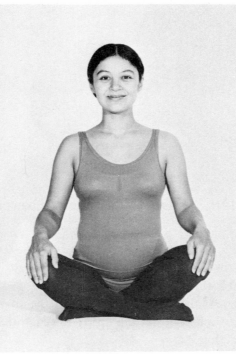

SUKHASANA (Easy Pose)

TECHNIQUE:

1. Sit on floor with legs crossed, hands resting on knees.
2. Back and neck are in one line with spine straight.
3. Eyes may be closed or focused on one spot in the distance. Breathing is normal.

BENEFITS: The benefits for Sukhasana, Ardha-Padmasana, Padmasana, and most cross-legged postures are the same. These exercises strengthen the muscles of the thighs and legs and enhance circulation while the ankle, knee, and hip joints are made flexible. The pelvis gets a new flow of blood and the stretch is most beneficial to the legs and lower back. Through practice of these Asanas, correct posture is maintained. Cross-legged postures are also emotionally relaxing.

ASWINI-MUDRA (Perineal Exercise)

TECHNIQUE:
1. Sit comfortably in a cross-legged position or sit on your heels in Vajrasana (Fixed Firm Pose, page 76).
2. Inhale and exhale. At the same time, contract the sphincter muscles (the circular muscles which contract the anus) drawing them in as though to prevent a bowel action.
3. Hold contraction to count of 5. Relax. Inhale again and repeat exercise. The movement should be a contraction while exhaling, relaxation while inhaling.
4. Gradually increase rapidity of contractions, inhaling to count of 4 while relaxing, exhaling to count of 4 while contracting, inhaling to count of 3 while relaxing, exhaling to count of 3 while contracting and so on until you are inhaling and exhaling to a steady count of 1 beat for each contracting and 1 beat for each relaxing movement.
5. This Mudra may be continued for 1 or 2 minutes. Once mastered, Perineal Exercise may be done as often as every 2 hours during the day. Perineal Exercise may be done in a standing position unobtrusively at odd times and at odd places: while washing dishes, waiting for a bus or a stoplight, almost anyplace!

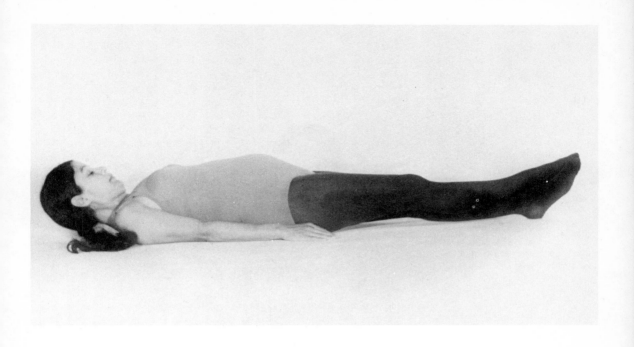

VARIATION FOR ASWINI-MUDRA

TECHNIQUE:

1. Lie on your back with ankles crossed.

2. Tilt pelvis pressing small of back against floor.

3. Squeeze thighs and pinch buttocks. Tighten up perineum (urinary and bowel passages) as if to hold back urination; then tighten up still higher inside vagina. Hold for count of 5. Repeat.

BENEFITS: *This is the most important exercise a woman can do before, during, and after pregnancy.* It is taught in natural-childbirth classes and is recommended by doctors. It massages and tones up female sex organs, including the vagina, and benefits the nerves and organs of the reproductive system. Practice of this Mudra increases elasticity of the pelvic floor muscles and helps to restore muscle function after delivery. It is recommended as an aid to eliminating bladder symptoms due to relaxation of the pelvic muscles, and is helpful in the prevention of both constipation and hemorrhoids. This Mudra may be done as a post-natal exercise in an inverted or semi-inverted posture for increased effectiveness in preventing or curing hemorrhoids. Aswini-Mudra also increases sexual proficiency and pleasure. This exercise is extremely beneficial and should become a part of every woman's life.

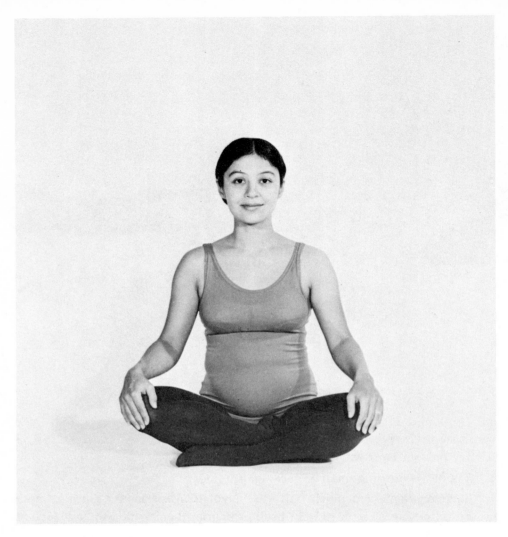

SIDDHASANA (Success in Meditation Pose)

TECHNIQUE:

1. Sit with left foot close to body, left knee bent.

2. Place right foot between left calf and thigh.

3. Spine is straight throughout. Hands rest on knees. Hold pose 20 seconds. Change sides.

4. Place right foot close to body and place left foot between right thigh and calf. Hold 20 seconds.

BENEFITS: See Sukhasana.

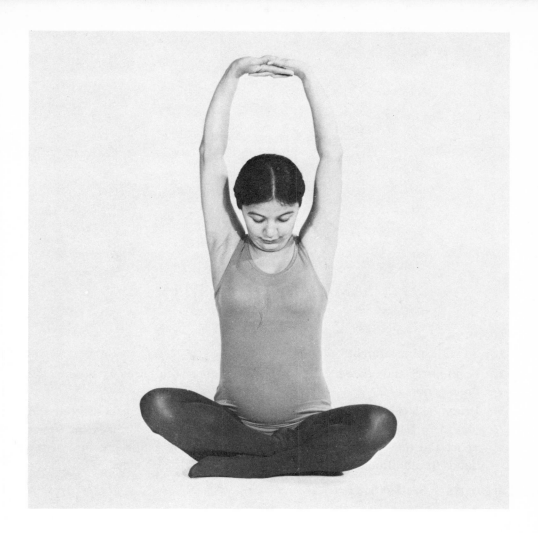

VARIATION FOR SIDDHASANA
(Success in Meditation Pose)

TECHNIQUE:

1. Sit in Siddhasana with spine straight, eyes closed. (See Siddhasana Technique.) Tuck chin into notch between collarbone.

2. Interlock fingers turning palms away from the body.

3. Keeping elbows as straight as possible (elbows will bend slightly), inhale to count of 5 while raising arms directly over the head.

4. Without pausing and retaining the breath, exhale slowly and smoothly to count of 5 and return hands to original position.

5. Repeat 6 times. Rest in position.

SAMASANA (Plain Pose)

TECHNIQUE:

1. Sit with spine straight.

2. Bend knees and place legs one before the other with knees as close to the floor as possible.

3. Bring the left heel close to the body; then place the right heel in front and almost in line with the left heel. (This automatically spreads the knees apart and they can be eased closer to the floor by gentle pressure of the hands for additional stretch.) Hold for 20 seconds each side.

BENEFITS: See Sukhasana.

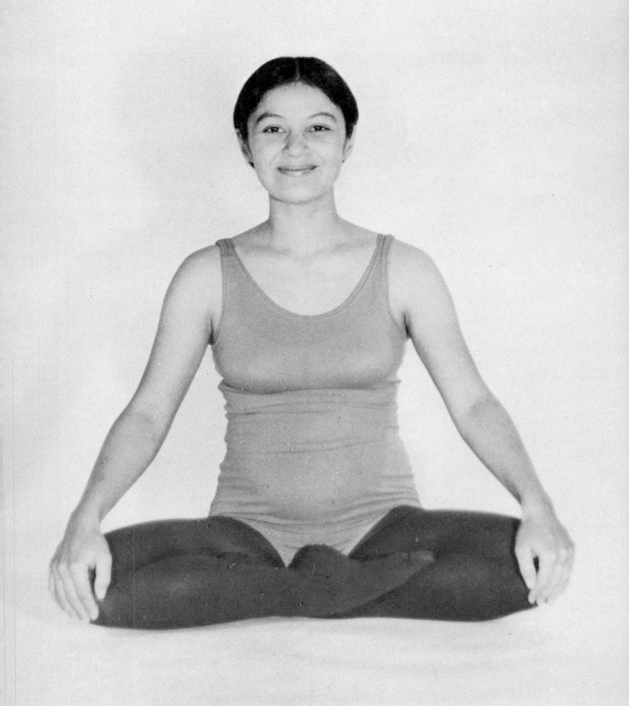

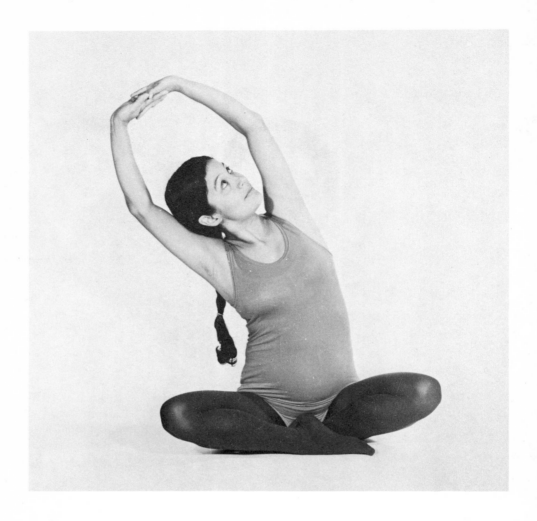

VARIATION FOR SAMASANA (Plain Pose)

TECHNIQUE:

1. Sit in Samasana with spine erect, eyes open.
2. Interlock fingers and turn palms away from the body.
3. Inhale to count of 5 and slowly raise arms above head.
4. Exhale to count of 5 and slowly bend body with arms extended above head to the right while turning the head up toward the ceiling. Take care not to twist the body and try to keep both knees on the floor.

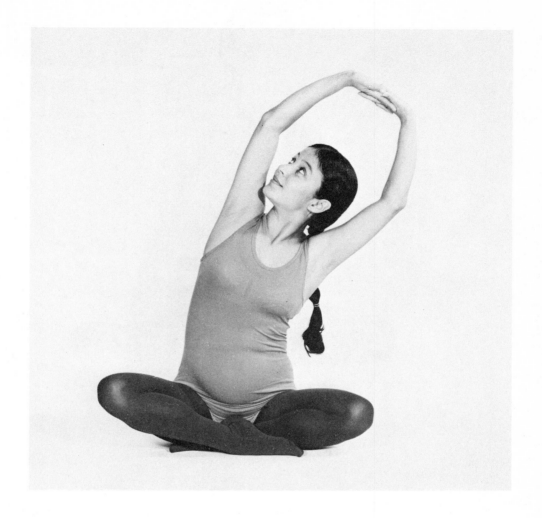

5. Inhale to count of 5 and return to upright position with arms above head, turning the head so you are facing the front.

6. Exhale to count of 5 and slowly bend body to the left, again turning head so you are looking straight up to the ceiling.

7. Inhale to count of 5 and return to upright position.

8. Exhale and lower hands to starting position. Repeat 4 times. Rest in position.

NOTE: May also be done in Siddhasana (Success in Meditation Pose).

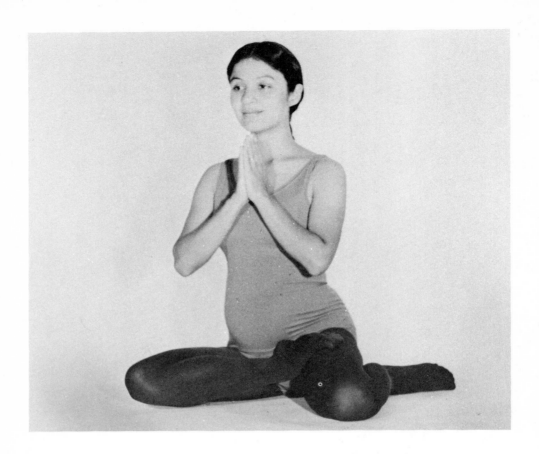

VIRASANA (Hero Pose)

TECHNIQUE:

1. Sit with spine straight. Starting with right leg, bend the knee **and bring** the leg close to the side of the body so that the knee points **forward and** the foot is toward the back.

2. Raise the left foot and rest it in Half Lotus position on the right thigh.

3. Hold 20 seconds. Change sides and hold for 20 seconds. Rest in position.

BENEFITS: See Sukhasana.

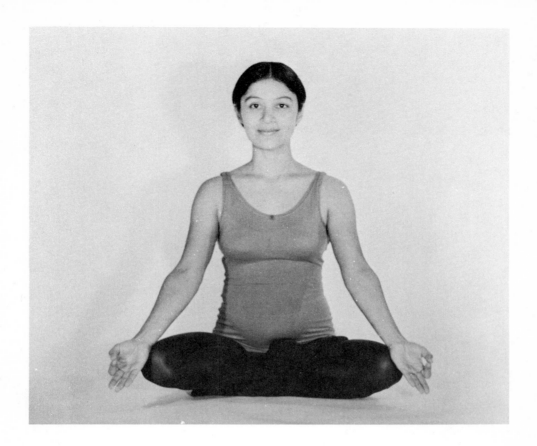

ARDHA-PADMASANA (Half Lotus Pose)

TECHNIQUE:

1. Sit erect stretching both legs forward.
2. Lift the right thigh, bending the knee, and place the left foot underneath.
3. Lift the right leg so that the right heel rests on the left thigh. (Heel should come close to the abdomen.)
4. Hands may either rest on knees, palms down, or palms up with thumb and forefinger forming a circle in traditional Yoga pose.
5. Hold 20 seconds. Alternate legs and again hold 20 seconds.
6. Gently stretch legs forward and vibrate knees. Rest.

BENEFITS: See Sukhasana.

NOTE: Only assume this posture if it is comfortable for you. Discontinue if it becomes difficult as pregnancy progresses.

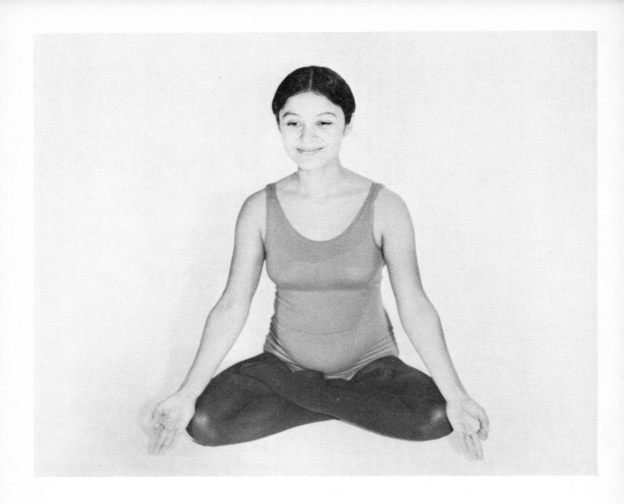

PADMASANA (Lotus Pose)

TECHNIQUE:

1. Sit in Sukhasana (Easy Pose) with spine straight.
2. Place right foot on left thigh with heel close to groin.
3. Place left foot on top of right thigh with heel close to groin.
4. Knees should be touching the floor or as close to the floor as possible.
5. Hands may press gently down on knees or rest palms up in traditional Lotus gesture. Hold 20 seconds.
6. Slowly stretch legs in front and vibrate knees.

BENEFITS: See Sukhasana. This posture provides maximum stretch in the leg and thigh muscles and helps to strengthen the muscles used in delivery.

NOTE: If this posture is too difficult, substitute one of the more comfortable cross-legged poses. Remember, never strain!

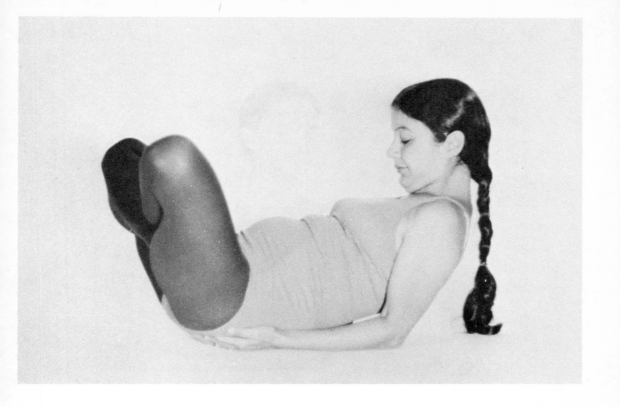

TULANGALASANA
(Lotus in "L" Shape on Back)

TECHNIQUE:

1. Assume Lotus Pose.
2. Place both hands under hips with palms cupping buttocks.
3. Gently lean back on your elbows without straining.
4. Legs are locked in the Lotus position and will raise up as you let yourself back. The body should form a 90° angle in an "L" shape with the legs in Lotus position forming the base of the "L".
5. Hold 20 seconds. Slowly relax legs and sit up *using the hands for support*.
6. Rest in position.

BENEFITS: If done with care, this posture provides soothing relaxation by counteracting the force of gravity and temporarily relieving the tension in the muscles supporting the weight of the baby.

NOTE: This posture should be attempted ONLY if the Lotus position is comfortable to assume.

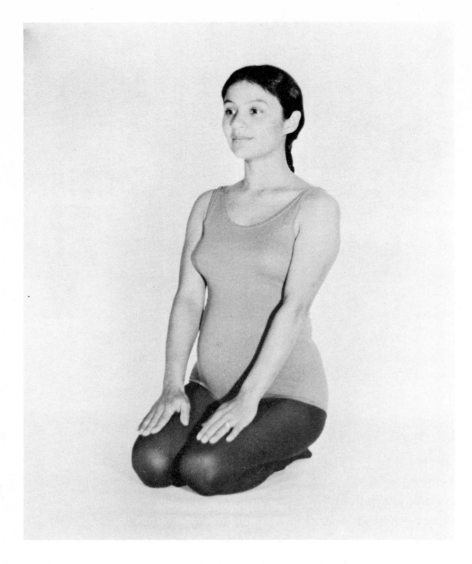

VAJRASANA (Fixed Firm Pose)

TECHNIQUE:

1. Kneel and sit on the feet with soles facing upward.

2. Keep knees together and place palms of hands on knees.

3. Keep spine perfectly straight, breathe normally, and hold position for 20 seconds.

BENEFITS: Aids digestion and removal of flatulence. Loosens and limbers up knee joints. Helps improve posture, an important aid during pregnancy. Also relieves cramps in toes, calves, knees, and thighs.

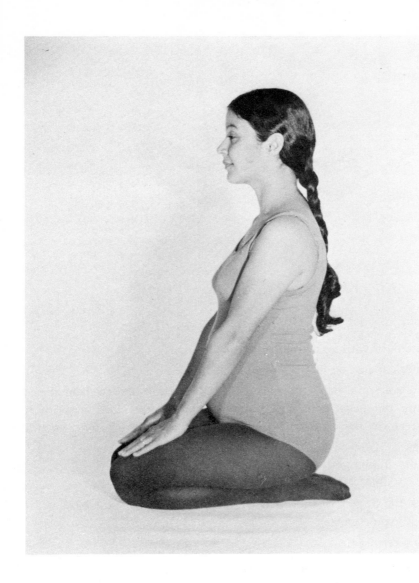

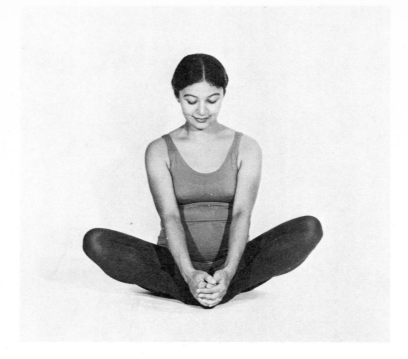

KONASANA (Angle Pose)

TECHNIQUE:

1. Sit on the floor with legs stretched out in front.

2. Bend knees and bring feet close to the body.

3. Bring the soles and heels of the feet together. Catch the feet near the toes and bring the heels near the perineum. The outer sides of both feet should rest on the floor and the back of the heels should touch the perineum.

4. Widen the thighs and lower the knees until they touch the floor or as close as possible.

5. Interlock the fingers of the hands, grip the feet firmly, and gaze straight ahead with spine erect.

6. Hold 20 seconds. Rest.

BENEFITS: Stretches and limbers up pelvic joints, perineal, and inner thigh muscles. Also counteracts the weight of the uterus which tends to pull the spine forward as pregnancy progresses, causing backache.

NOTE: This is how the Indian cobblers sit. This Asana is excellent for strengthening the pelvic muscles and the small of the back and will reduce labor pains considerably if practiced regularly. Try to spend 10 to 15 minutes a day in this pose.

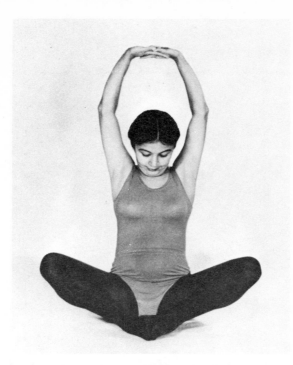

BADDHA-KONASANA (Bound Angle Pose)

TECHNIQUE:

1. Sit on the floor in Konasana with soles of feet touching, knees close to the floor.

2. After assuming this position, interlock fingers with palms away from the body touching heels, rest chin in notch between collarbone, and close your eyes.

3. Inhale to count of 5 and slowly raise arms with interlocked hands above head.

4. Exhale to count of 5 and slowly lower arms to starting position—with hands touching heels.

5. Repeat 4 times. Rest in Konasana with eyes closed.

6. Grasp toes lightly with interlocked fingers.

7. Take 4 deep breaths in this position, inhaling and exhaling to count of 5.

8. Rest in Savasana.

BENEFITS: Stretches and limbers up pelvic joints, perineal, and inner thigh muscles as it increases circulation to the breasts and strengthens the pectoral muscles which support them. Elevates the diaphragm and rib cage while affording more room in the abdomen. May relieve heartburn and indigestion.

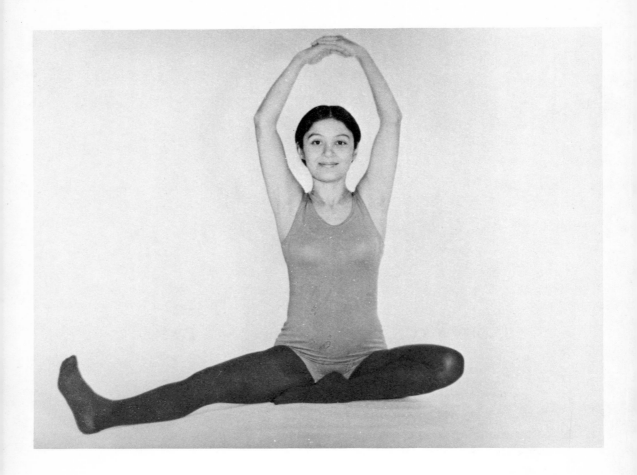

MAHA-MUDRA (Great Mudra)

TECHNIQUE:

1. Sit with spine erect and extend right leg straight ahead.
2. Draw left leg up to body until sole of left foot rests against right thigh, heel touching perineum.
3. Tuck chin in notch between collarbone. Eyes may be closed for greater relaxation.
4. Lightly cup hands with left hand resting in right.
5. Inhale to count of 5 raising arms with hands cupped above head.

HEALTHY PREGNANCY THE YOGA WAY

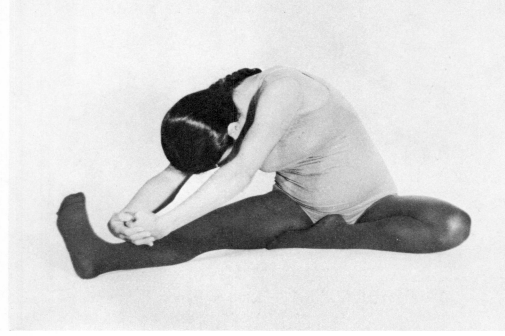

6. Exhale to count of 5 bending forward over right leg and bring hands to rest on shin about 2 inches below the knee with left hand resting palm down on shin bone and right hand on top of left.

7. Remain in this position with shoulders relaxed and take 6 breaths, inhaling and exhaling to count of 5.

8. Inhale and return to sitting position with arms extended above head. Exhale slowly, lowering arms to starting position.

9. Rest 20 seconds. Change sides and repeat.

10. Rest in Savasana.

BENEFITS: This is a gentle Asana conducive to relaxation. Also tones up circulation and increases oxygen intake while aiding breath control.

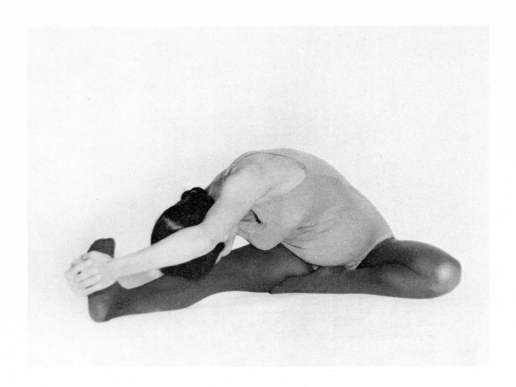

JANUSHIRASANA (Head to Knee Pose)

TECHNIQUE:

1. Sit with spine straight and legs extended in front of the body.
2. Bend left knee and place left heel up to beginning of right thigh.
3. Slide right leg out to a 45° angle away from the body.
4. Interlock fingers of both hands, inhale, and raise hands above the head.
5. Exhale and bend forward over the right leg as far down as is comfortable. Try to catch behind your toes. Hold 10 seconds.
6. Change sides and repeat. Rest in Savasana.

BENEFITS: May aid in prevention and relief of indigestion and constipation. Strengthens legs and bladder support thereby improving bladder function.

NOTE: It is important not to strain in this posture. The hands may catch the toes or come to rest anywhere on the shin. Always stop before reaching the point of strain.

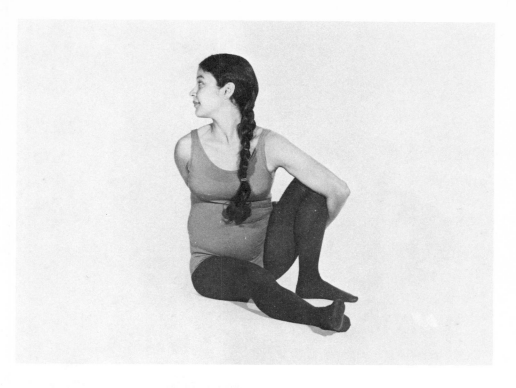

ARDHA-MATSYENDRASANA
(Spine Twisting Pose)
Modified Variation for Pregnancy

TECHNIQUE:

1. Sit on the floor with both legs extended in front.

2. Bend right knee. Lean forward and catch the right knee with the inside elbow of the right arm. Right hand will be on the outside of the leg.

3. Firmly anchor pelvic region and bring left arm around back of the body, turning the head to look over the left (rear) shoulder.

4. Try to lock hands behind you while gently twisting the body to accommodate pose. Straighten spine and hold 20 seconds.

5. Change sides extending right leg and bending left knee. Hold 20 seconds.

6. Rest in Savasana.

BENEFITS: Circulation is increased while lungs are expanded and become more flexible. Both upper and lower back are stretched and made more flexible while the deep muscles of the spine are strengthened. Practice of this Asana corrects poor posture and counteracts obesity, constipation, and indigestion resulting from poor posture and lack of exercise.

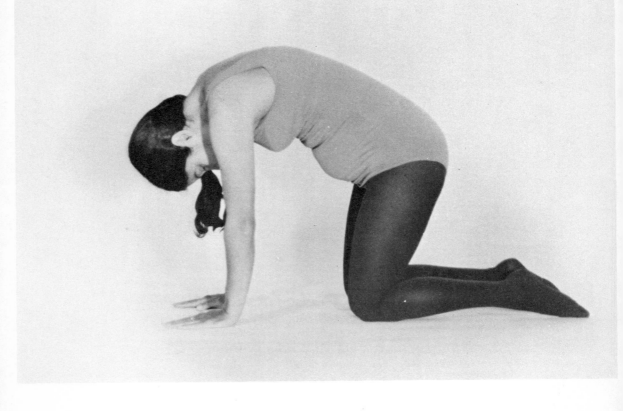

BIDALASANA (The Cat)

TECHNIQUE:

1. Kneel with hands on the floor directly below the shoulders, knees below the hips, head hanging down.

2. Inhale to count of 5. Exhale to count of 5 and manipulate spine by raising it to form an arch in the back (spine is humped up).

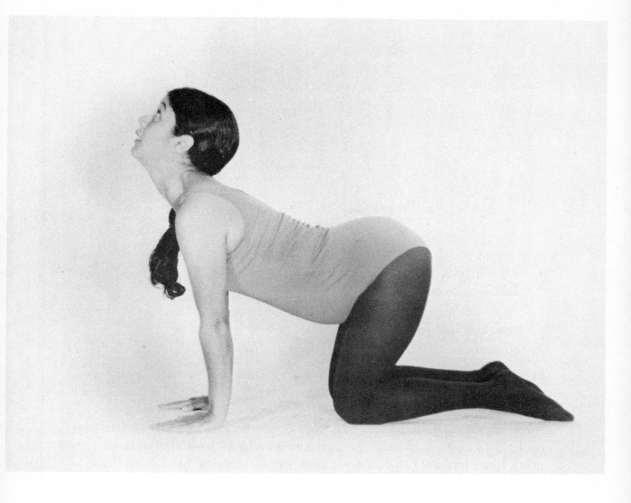

3. Inhale to count of 5 and raise face toward the ceiling while relaxing the back, forming a deep depression in the spine.

4. Exhale to count of 5 as you hump back. Inhale to count of 5 as you raise head and depress back.

5. Repeat for 6 breaths.

6. Rest in Savasana.

BENEFITS: This position allows the abdominal organs to hang from the posterior abdominal wall relieving the pressure usually exerted by the force of gravity as they fall toward the pelvis, pressing on the great blood vessels and the nerves. Limbers and loosens the joints of the spine, lower pelvis, and hips, and strengthens the abdominal muscles. Improves posture and alleviates or prevents backache. This is an extremely important Asana to practice during pregnancy.

VARIATION FOR BIDALASANA (The Cat)

TECHNIQUE:

1. Lie on back in Savasana and press the small of the back to the floor. Inhale to count of 5.

2. Arch the back, keeping hips and shoulders on the floor, and exhale to count of 5.

3. Repeat 6 times. Rest.

BENEFITS: These exercises are most important for comfort during pregnancy. Practice of these Asanas increases the flexibility of the lower back, strengthens abdominal muscles, and shifts your center of gravity toward the spine improving your posture and your appearance (especially in late pregnancy). There is an added benefit in that learning to stand and walk with the pelvis tilted forward provides your baby with a cradle of bone in which to lie and thereby avoids further stretching of the abdominal wall.

CHAPTER

6

SPECIAL PROBLEMS
THAT MAY ARISE
DURING PREGNANCY

Yoga Can Help the Natural Way

Fetal development is accompanied by extensive changes in the mother's body make-up and metabolism. As your body undergoes these physiological changes, you may or may not be bothered with some of the common problems associated with having a baby. Gastric tone, motility, and secretion are reduced, often causing nausea, heartburn, and constipation. There are many Yogasanas and *sattvic* (pure) foods that may be effective in combating the annoyance of leg cramps, constipation, varicose veins, flatulence, and backache without resorting to drugs, medicines, or other artificial means of control. Always consult your physician concerning *any* problem you may have during pregnancy and follow his advice.

Nausea or Morning Sickness

Nausea or morning sickness, most common during the first months of pregnancy, is seldom confined to mornings and may strike at any time during the day or night. It is comforting to know that morning sickness usually disappears by the end of the third month. In the meantime, it helps to eat five or six small meals a day to keep the stomach from being empty; smaller meals are also easier to digest. Eat without drinking liquids and take them between meals instead. Avoid rich, fatty foods and strong spices and forget butter and fried foods; you probably won't be hungry for them anyway.

Carbohydrates are easy to digest and seem to be better tolerated than other foods early in pregnancy; it may help to nibble on a few dry crackers when feeling nauseated. Soda crackers are traditional! Try eating breakfast in bed with a carbohydrate tray of crackers or toast, honey, and cold cereal. Carbohydrates also provide quick energy, iron, roughage, and B vitamins. Vitamin B_1 or B_6 has been found to help in cases of nausea but should be prescribed by your doctor, as should any vitamin. You may eat natural foods rich in B vitamins, however, and good snack foods containing high quantities of B vitamins include bananas, raw pecans, and wheat germ. Fortified brewer's yeast, sprouted mung beans, and lentils are also high in B vitamins.

It may help to rest in Savasana for 20 minutes following each meal. However, if you suffer from heartburn (a mild form of indigestion), it's best not to lie down immediately after eating.

Heartburn

Heartburn (gastric reflux) during pregnancy is caused by internal crowding as the baby grows and takes up more room. If heartburn strikes, don't sit or lie down to rest but get up and move about. If you feel that burning sensation in your chest, stand up and perform two sets of Deep Breathing. This will expand your rib cage, giving your digestive system more room in which to function, and help to relieve the condition. Stay away from baking soda as this is not recommended during pregnancy. Eating at least a half cup of yogurt a day aids digestion.

That Common Backache

Almost all pregnant women complain at some time during their pregnancy of varying degrees of back pain. This is due to postural change related to the growth of the baby which causes increased lumbar lordosis which, in turn, may cause lower back pain. There is also a temporary relaxation of the vagina and pelvis during pregnancy which causes greater stress on the lumbo-sacral joints, again resulting in lower backache.

To combat backaches, wear low heeled shoes to give you better balance. Be aware of your posture and consciously correct it during the day by practicing the Pelvic Tilt. If your back begins to pain you, lie down in Savasana and get as much rest as you can.

The following Asanas provide relief and are a real help in preventing backache, when regularly practiced:

1. *Bidalasana (The Cat) and Variations:* This is one of the best postures for relieving backache.

2. *Devipadapeetham (The Bridge Pose):* This Asana is also excellent for relieving and preventing lower back pain.

3. *Ardha-Chandrasana (Half Moon Pose)*

4. *Janushirasana (Head to Knee Pose)*

5. *Ardha-Matsyendrasana (Spine Twisting Pose)*

Varicose Veins

Varicose veins are enlarged leg veins that lie just beneath the skin. The added weight gain of pregnancy sometimes puts enough added pressure on the legs to aggravate this condition. Resting in Savasana frequently during the day with your feet propped up between 14 to 20 inches helps. Your doctor may prescribe wearing elastic stockings during the day. Keep them on your bedside table and put them on before you get up in the morning so the leg veins won't have a chance to fill up.

Vitamin C and the bioflavonoids (vitamin P) help strengthen capillary walls and also help to avert toxemia. These are found in the white membranes of citrus fruits and in green peppers and potatoes. A tasty natural beverage worth trying is the Lemon Drink.

LEMON DRINK

1 thick-skinned lemon
3 vitamin C tablets
2 to 3 tablespoons honey
1 cup water

Thinly peel the lemon, leaving as much white membrane as possible, and remove the seeds. Add water, vitamin C tablets, and honey to taste. Whip in a blender for 3 minutes. Use as a base for Lemon Drink by adding 2 tbsp. to a glass of water. Drink frequently during the day.

Regular practice of Garurasana (Eagle Pose) is an aid to this condition during pregnancy. All inverted postures are excellent as post-natal Asanas to combat varicose veins. Halasana (Plough Pose) and Sarvangasana (Shoulder Stand) should be practiced at least twice a day *after* the baby is born. Supta-Vajrasana is effective as a post-natal Asana.

Hemorrhoids (Piles)

Hemorrhoids are groups of enlarged blood vessels located at the lower end of the bowel. Obstruction of venous blood return to the heart due to pressure on the inferior vena cava by the enlarged uterus may contribute to the development of hemorrhoids. Good bowel habits help to prevent hemorrhoids. Try to avoid straining during bowel movements. A little petroleum jelly placed just inside the rectum may help. Hot sitz baths afford temporary relief and are helpful in treating hemorrhoids.

The strain of childbirth may cause hemorrhoids to be a post-natal problem. Practice of Aswini-Mudra in Vipareeta-Karani (Perineal Exercise in Half-shoulder Stand) has effected amazing results in many cases of severe hemorrhoids. This Asana is highly recommended if hemorrhoids appear after the baby is born.

Aswini-Mudra in Vipareeta-Karani (Perineal Exercise in Half-shoulder Stand)

TECHNIQUE:
1. Lie in Savasana and slowly lift the legs and body up into a vertical position, supporting yourself by placing hands under the hips. Body weight will be on the elbows and upper arms; body will be at an angle of about 30° from the vertical.
2. Hold this pose and perform Aswini-Mudra by alternately tightening and relaxing the sphincter muscles and the muscles around the vagina. Practice Aswini-Mudra 30 times with normal breathing. This will take some practice, but the condition *will improve* and often disappear through regular performance of this Asana.
3. Slowly lower legs and return to Savasana. Relax. Perform several times daily.

Leg Cramps

Women sometimes suffer from cramps in the feet and legs during pregnancy, often while resting or in the middle of the night. Lack of calcium can be a cause of cramping. Sometimes the increase of milk in the diet may result in an excess of phosphorus which may lead to cramps, and your doctor may have you reduce or eliminate your milk intake and supplement the milk's nutrients with other foods. The sodium content in milk may also cause a fluid weight gain which may result in leg cramps. If you are troubled by a fluid weight gain or water retention in the body, reduce or eliminate salt and salty foods. Your doctor may approve the use of natural diuretics which are better for you than water pills.

Natural diuretics include cranberry juice, coffee, and special tisanes (herb teas) such as Corn Silk Tea, Meadow-Sweet Tea, Cherry Stems Tea, and Horse Tail Tea. Prepare a fresh pot of tea daily and drink at least four full cups alone (not with meals) during the day. Flavor with honey, lemon, or mint if desired. Solid foods that may act as natural diuretics include asparagus, watercress, grapefruit, apples, radishes, grapes, and pineapple.

Sodium exchange resins in some water softening systems add an enormous amount of salt to the water. If you have a home water softener, check with your dealer to be sure that it is not adding salt when removing other chemicals.

If you have a leg cramp or a cramp in your toes or feet, bend the affected part in the opposite direction of the cramp, holding with the hands if necessary, until the cramp disappears. Avoid pointing the toe. Point your heel, not your toe!

Problems Nobody Likes to Talk About: Constipation and Flatulence

Constipation is likely to occur both during pregnancy and after childbirth. *It is inadvisable to take laxatives during pregnancy.* Natural aids to elimination are relaxation, plenty of exercise, adequate fluids, and bulk in the diet. The best way to fight constipation is through a well-balanced diet and regular practice of Yogasanas. Tension contributes to constipation by constricting the muscles necessary for proper bowel functioning. Drinking a glass of tepid or warm water first thing in the morning aids elimination. Some people prefer to add lemon juice and honey, feeling this is even more effective.

Prune juice is the best natural laxative. Honey has laxative properties as do certain fruits such as cooked dried prunes and fresh peaches, while bananas have a constipating effect. Other yogic foods with laxative properties are pure vegetable oils (corn oil, safflower oil, or wheat germ oil are delicious in salad dressings with raw green vegetables which provide necessary bulk in the diet), wheat germ itself (add it to breakfast cereals or fruit salads), molasses, yeast mixed with fruit or vegetable juices, and yogurt.

Try to have a regular time to move your bowels; after breakfast is a good time. Avoid straining. If the problem becomes severe, do ask your doctor for his advice.

Daily practice of your regular schedule of Yogasanas is the best pre-natal prevention for constipation. Post-natal Asanas effective in eliminating constipation are:

1. *Ardha-Chandrasana with Pada-Hastasana* (*Half Moon Pose with Hands to Feet Posture*)

2. *Janushirasana* (*Head to Knee Pose*)

3. *Dandayamana-Bibhaktapada-Paschimotthanasana* (*Standing Separate Leg Stretching Pose*)

4. *Ardha-Matsyendrasana* (*Spinal Twist*)

5. *Uddiyana-Bandha* (*Abdominal Contraction*)

6. *Nauli* (*The Churning Exercise*)

Uddiyana-Bandha and the Nauli are *not* to be practiced during pregnancy as they involve violent stomach contractions. However, they are extremely effective to banish constipation after the baby is born.

As the baby grows larger, the intestines are depressed by the added pressure from the uterus, causing flatulence or gas. The easiest and most effective ante-natal Asana for flatulence is simply to sit in Vajrasana (Fixed Firm Pose). This relieves the discomfort within minutes. Another way to achieve relief is to lie down on your left side with your top leg flexed and your bottom leg straight. This position helps direct the gas across the transverse colon to the descending colon where it may be readily expelled.

Avoid certain gas-forming foods during pregnancy as you may be particularly sensitive to them then. The best foods to avoid when troubled by flatulence are baked beans, broccoli, brussels sprouts, cabbage, cauliflower, cucumbers, onions, radishes, and turnips. Cooked sulfur foods, such as cabbage, cauliflower, eggs, peas, and beans, should never be combined with starches at a meal as this inevitably produces gas.

Post-natal Asanas recommended for flatulence are:

1. *Pavanamuktasana* (*Gas Removing Pose*)

2. *Bhujangasana Series* (*Cobra Series*) Including the Cobra, Half-Locust, Full-Locust, and Bow Poses.

Headaches

Tension headaches benefit from complete relaxation in Savasana. For continuing or severe headaches, consult your doctor immediately.

CHAPTER

7

POST-NATAL ASANAS

Post-partum Exercises to Start in Bed

There are many reasons for beginning a mild set of post-partum exercises as soon as you feel up to it. You will fit into your clothes faster, look better, and regain your energy more quickly if you begin to exercise while still in the hospital. Aswini-Mudra (Perineal Exercise), Deep Breathing, and the Pelvic Tilt may all be done in bed. These gentle exercises can hasten your recovery and you will feel better for doing them. Exercising after baby arrives also helps to relieve constipation, which is very common after childbirth. Low-back pain is also prevalent after delivery and exercising immediately can help to alleviate it. The following exercises may be done in bed:

1. *Aswini-Mudra (Perineal Exercise)*

    TECHNIQUE: Lie on your back, arms at your sides, knees straight and legs crossed at the ankles. Practice Aswini-Mudra by tightening the muscles of the hips and pelvic floor as if checking a bowel movement. Repeat 10 times twice daily for 2 days, then stop.

2. *Deep Breathing in Prone Posture*

    TECHNIQUE: Lie on your back, arms at your sides, knees straight, no pillow. Raise arms up over your head while inhaling to count of 5. At the same time, push your feet down as if standing on tip-toe. Exhale to count of 5 while bringing arms back to your sides and pull your feet up as if standing on your heels. Repeat 5 times twice daily for one week, then stop.

3. *Pelvic Tilt*

    TECHNIQUE: Lie on your back, arms at your sides, knees bent and feet flat, no pillow. Flatten back against the bed or floor by pulling the abdomen in and rolling hips upward. Repeat 10 times twice daily for one week, then stop.

Ease cramps in your feet and calves by bending your feet at the ankles, tensing, and then relaxing them. You may also rotate your feet in a circular motion, first to the right, then to the left and relax.

The following exercises may be started 3 days after childbirth:

1. *Head and Shoulder Raising*

> TECHNIQUE: Lie on your back, arms at your sides, knees bent, feet flat, no pillow. Place chin on chest, lift your head and shoulders off the bed or floor, and reach forward toward your knees. Slowly lower head and shoulders. Repeat 10 times twice daily for one week, then stop.

2. *Hip Lifting*

> TECHNIQUE: Lie on your back, arms at your sides, knees bent, feet flat and slightly apart, no pillow. Raise hips until your body rests only on your shoulders and feet. Press your knees together tightly and do Aswini-Mudra 10 times. Repeat twice daily for one week, then stop.

3. *Alternate Straight-leg Lowering*

> TECHNIQUE: Lie on your back, arms at your sides, legs straight, no pillow. Bring left knee to your chest and straighten leg toward the ceiling. Hold leg straight, keep back flat, and slowly lower leg. Repeat 10 times with each leg twice daily for 3 weeks, then stop.

Check with your doctor four weeks after the birth of your baby or during your post-partum appointment on the advisability of starting your post-natal Yoga program. If he approves, adapt the following Asanas to your own use for a rapid post-natal figure recovery program. You will be amazed at how quickly you will regain your figure through regular practice of these simple Yogasanas. Many of the postures included in the list of Ante-natal Asanas are also very effective in firming the abdomen, waistline, hips, and upper thighs.

Three Techniques to Tighten that Tummy

The major problem area of most concern to a new mother is her stomach. Abdominal muscles stretched from pregnancy and childbirth need time and exercise to regain their former elasticity and tone. Although the uterus is generally back in the pelvis two weeks after birth, it usually takes about six weeks for the uterus to shrink completely to its former size. Yogasanas aimed at strengthening abdominal muscles can help immensely. You can regain your figure and retain your energy level by following a regular exercise program. The following three Asanas are specifically aimed at tightening the tummy:

1. *Utthita-Padasana* (*Advanced Leg Lifting Pose*)

    TECHNIQUE: Lie in Savasana and clasp your hands behind your neck. Slowly raise both legs together until toes point straight up to the ceiling, both knees locked. Slowly lower legs until heels almost touch the floor but not quite. Again raise legs up to perpendicular, then lower. Repeat 5 times, slowly lower legs and rest in Savasana.

2. *Uddiyana-Bandha* (*Abdominal Contraction*)

    TECHNIQUE: In standing position, place feet about 12 inches apart, rest your hands on your thighs, and slightly bend your knees. Lean slightly forward with your weight on your hands, inhale deeply through the nose, and exhale *completely* through the mouth. Contract the abdominal muscles, drawing the stomach in as far as possible toward the spine. At the same time, raise the diaphragm. (The abdomen should form a deep hollow under the ribs.) Maintain position for as long as you can hold your breath comfortably without inhaling. Then relax and repeat the exercise. *Uddiyana-Bandha* may also be done in a cross-legged position.

NOTE: Uddiyana-Bandha is of special importance to women as the abdominal contractions affect and stimulate the sex glands, the uterus, and the entire reproductive system thereby helping to aid menstrual disorders. *Never practice Uddiyana-Bandha during menstruation or pregnancy.* Practice only on an empty stomach, preferably first thing in the morning. Regular practice of Uddiyana-Bandha and the Nauli is effective in eliminating constipation.

3. *Nauli* (*Churning Exercise*)

    TECHNIQUE: Uddiyana-Bandha must be mastered before the Nauli is attempted. This may take some time and practice, but is well worth the effort involved. In the Nauli, the abdominal muscles are manipulated in a rhythmical manner by first contracting, then relaxing the muscles in a rotary flapping movement. Try to make a *forward* and *downward* thrusting movement with your stomach muscles by rotating them in rapid succession. With practice, you can learn to isolate the two oblique muscles of the abdomen which run from the ribs to the pubic bone. They will stand out quite clearly when the exercise is practiced correctly. Practice in front of a mirror until you become proficient. Repeat 3 times and relax.

All forward-stretching Asanas are good as any forward bending of the spine vigorously contracts the abdominal muscles. Backward-bending motions also exercise and strengthen the abdominal wall. These Asanas are also effective in toning the abdominal area:

1. *The Boat* (*Head and Leg Lifting Pose*)

2. *Pavanamuktasana* (*Gas Removing Pose*)

3. *Janushirasana with Paschimotthanasana* (*Sitting Head to Knee Pose with Stretching Posture*)

4. *Halasana* (*Plough Pose*)

5. *Sit-ups from Savasana*

6. *Ardha-Kurmasana* (*Half Tortoise Pose*)

7. *Bhujangasana* (*Cobra*)

8. *Salabhasana* (*Locust Pose*)

9. *Poorna-Salabhasana* (*Full Locust Pose*)

10. *Dhanurasana* (*Bow Pose*)

Spot Asanas for Waistline, Hips, and Under Thighs

Aside from the abdomen, other problem areas which concern new mothers are the waistline, hips, and upper thighs, all of which seem to have a way of expanding following childbirth. Asanas recommended for stomach firming are also helpful in trimming inches from the waist with twisting postures proving especially effective. All cross-legged postures are good for firming thighs while backward bending poses benefit hips and buttocks. The following Asanas are recommended for these specific areas:

For the Waistline:

1. *Ardha-Chandrasana with Pada-Hastasana (Half Moon Pose with Hands to Feet Posture)*: This is a superb exercise for slimming the waistline.

2. *Janushirasana with Paschimotthanasana (Sitting Head to Knee Pose with Stretching Posture)*

3. *Gomukhasana (Cow Face Pose)*

4. *Halasana (Plough Pose)*

5. *Bhujangasana (Cobra Pose)*

6. *Dhanurasana (Bow Pose)*

7. *Poorna-Salabhasana (Full Locust Pose)*

For the Hips and Upper Thighs:

1. All Cross-legged Postures, especially *Konasana*

2. *Ardha-Matsyendrasana (Spinal Twist)*

3. *Halasana (Plough Pose)*

4. *Utkatasana (Awkward Sitting Pose)*: Especially effective for reducing inches from the thigh.

5. *Garurasana (Eagle Pose)*: Also good for reducing the thigh.

6. *Dhanurasana (Bow Pose)*

7. *Salabhasana (Locust Pose)*

NOTE: For quick results, perform the specific Asanas recommended for the problem areas with which you are concerned both in the morning and at night or at odd times during the day, apart from your regular exercise period. Persistence pays off!

SUGGESTED PRACTICE SCHEDULE
OF POST-NATAL ASANAS
(TO BEGIN FOUR WEEKS AFTER BIRTH)

Prone Postures

TECHNIQUES AND BENEFITS
FOR
STANDING, SITTING, AND PRONE POSTURES

DEEP-BREATHING ASANA

TECHNIQUE:

1. Stand with feet together and spine erect. Clasp hands, under chin, fingers interlocked, and palms together.

2. Inhale deeply through the nostrils with mouth closed while raising elbows toward the ceiling. Fingers remain locked while palms separate. Hands touch chin at all times.

3. Exhale through the throat passage with mouth open, bringing elbows together as you push your head back.

4. Inhale while bringing head slowly down to starting position, again raising elbows. (By raising your arms to the sides, you automatically expand the rib cage allowing the lungs to fill completely with air.)

5. Repeat for 10 breaths. Eyes remain open throughout or dizziness may occur.

6. Rest with arms relaxed at sides for 20 seconds. Repeat a second set.

BENEFITS: This Asana should always be done before beginning any exercise session as it awakens the body by increasing the general circulation and flooding the lungs with life-giving oxygen.

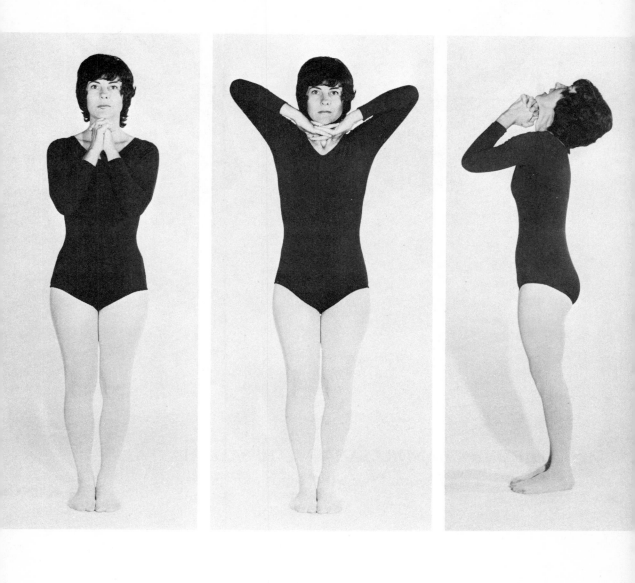

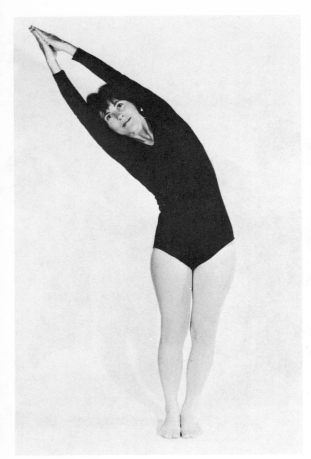 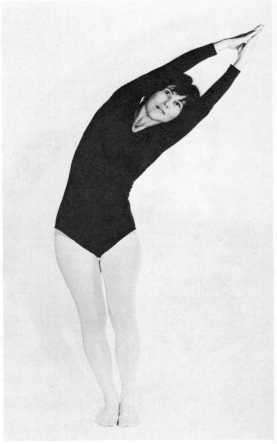

ARDHA-CHANDRASANA WITH PADA-HASTASANA
(Half Moon Pose with Hands to Feet Posture)

TECHNIQUE:

1. Stand erect with feet together. Slowly raise arms sidewise above head until palms are together in Namascar.

2. Stretch up toward the ceiling and bend to the right without twisting the body. Hold for count of 10.

3. Slowly straighten position, stretch up and bend to the left. Hold for count of 10.

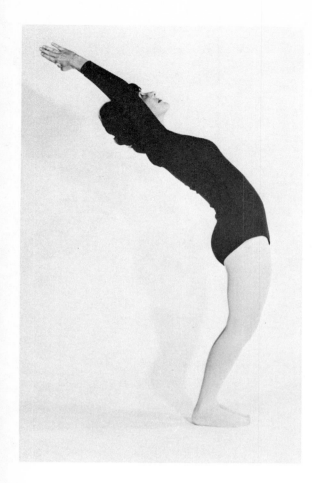
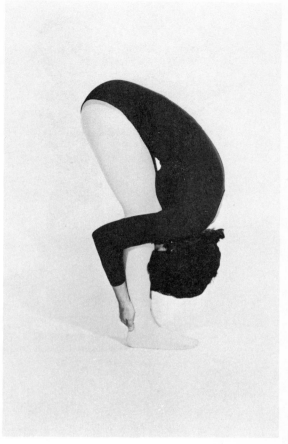

4. Straighten position. Drop head all the way back and push the stomach forward bringing arms to the rear as far as possible. Hold for count of 10.

5. Straighten position. Inhale deeply. Exhale and bend forward, arms and head together. Grab the back of your ankles with both hands and touch the forehead to the knees, keeping the knees locked. If you cannot touch your knees, go down as far as you can, grab the back of your legs, and hold for count of 10.

6. Come up with arms and head together. Slowly lower arms to the sides and relax. Repeat a second set.

BENEFITS: Strengthens the abdominal wall and tightens stomach muscles. Firms and trims the waistline.

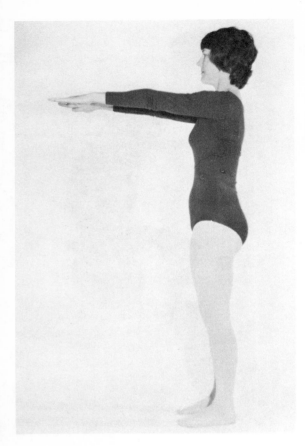 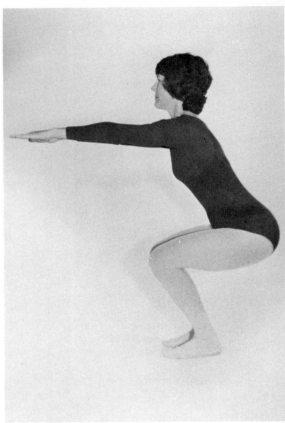

UTKATASANA (Awkward Sitting Pose)

TECHNIQUE:

1. Stand erect with feet flat on the floor 6 inches apart. Raise both arms in front until parallel to the floor, palms facing down. Slowly bend knees keeping feet flat on the floor until thighs are parallel to the floor. (Imagine yourself sitting in a straight-backed chair.) Hold for 10 seconds. Straighten to standing position.

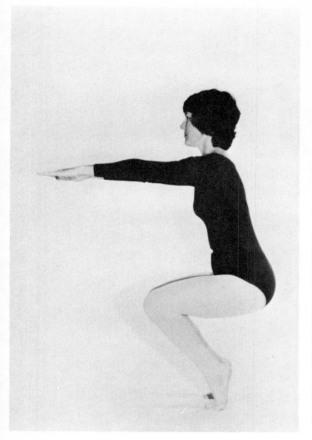 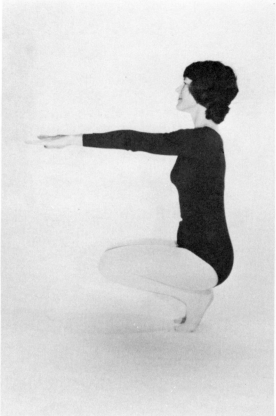

2. Keeping arms extended, raise up on the toes and slowly bend knees to sitting position while keeping your balance. Again, thighs should be parallel to the floor. Hold 10 seconds, straighten to standing position and relax feet, arms still outstretched.

3. Raise up on the toes once more and slowly bend, knees together, until you are sitting on your heels. Hold 10 seconds. Slowly straighten to standing position with feet flat on the floor and lower arms to the sides. Relax in standing posture. Repeat a second set.

BENEFITS: Firms the upper arms. Especially good for tightening hips, calves, and upper thighs. This Asana has been known to change a 32″ thigh to a 22″ thigh over a period of time.

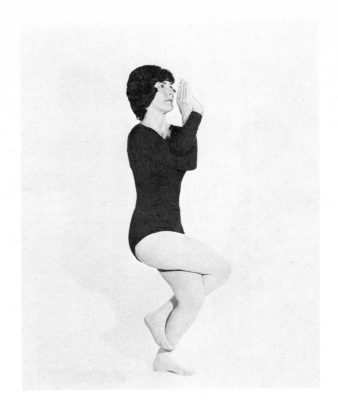

GARURASANA (Eagle Pose)

TECHNIQUE:

1. Wrap right arm under left arm at elbow and place palms together with thumbs crossed in Namascar.

2. Balance on left foot and wrap right leg over left leg, crossing at thigh. Bend knees to accommodate posture and hook right foot behind left calf. Thigh should be parallel to the floor.

3. Straighten spine while maintaining balance and tighten posture. Hold for 10 seconds.

4. Unwind and change sides.

5. Wrap left arm under right arm. Balance on right foot and wrap left leg over right, hooking left foot around right calf. Tighten and hold 10 seconds.

6. Unwind and rest in standing position. Repeat.

BENEFITS: Tightens upper thighs, abdomen, and upper arms. Stimulates sex glands. Helps prevent varicose veins.

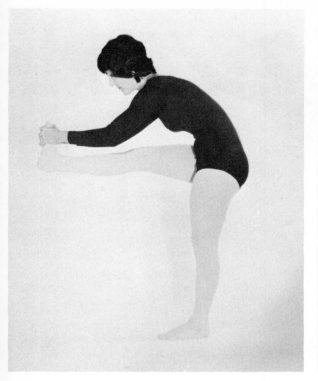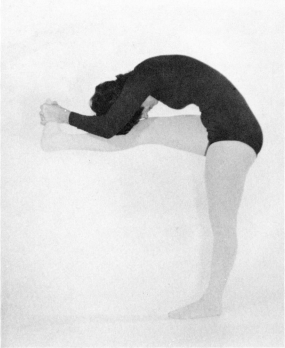

DANDAYAMANA-JANUSHIRASANA
(Standing Head to Knee Pose)

TECHNIQUE:

1. Stand erect with left knee locked. (It is important to lock the knee of the leg you are standing on as this assures balance in any standing posture.) Raise the right leg and catch the toes with interlocked fingers of both hands. Slowly straighten right leg while keeping your balance.

2. When you are steady, continue to grip the toes and slowly drop the forehead to touch the right knee. Hold for 10 seconds. Eyes must be open to maintain balance.

3. Slowly straighten posture, bend right knee, and release.

4. Change sides, balancing on right leg and raising left leg. Both knees should be straight. (This is a difficult pose to master and takes some practice.) Rest in standing position. Repeat pose.

BENEFITS: Helps to tighten abdominal muscles and those of the upper thigh. An excellent posture for developing balance.

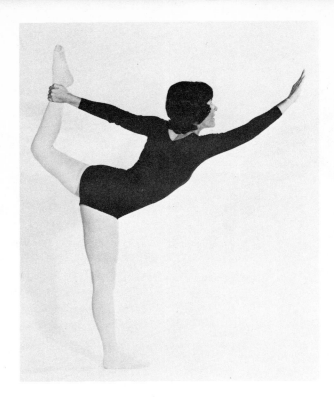

DANDAYAMANA-DHANURASANA
(Standing Bow Pose)

TECHNIQUE:

1. Balance on the left leg with left knee locked. Catch inside right ankle with right hand in a firm grip with thumb and fingers together, thumb toward ceiling.

2. Stretch left arm out in front of the body with fingers extended in a straight line pointing upward at a 45° angle.

3. Gradually bend forward with left arm extended and slowly kick back and up with the right foot, toe pointed. Hold for 10 seconds.

4. Relax and change sides. Hold left leg while balancing on right leg and kick back and up. Hold 10 seconds.

5. Relax in standing position. Repeat pose.

BENEFITS: Firms the abdominal wall and tightens upper thighs. Firms upper arms, hips, and buttocks. Dandayamana-Dhanurasana is the reverse posture of Dandayamana-Janushirasana and should always follow it. Yoga strives for harmony and balance; hence, a forward-bending posture is usually followed by a backward-bending pose.

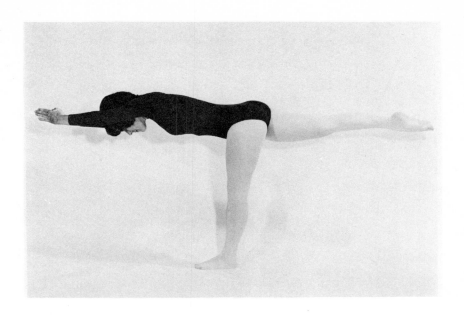

TULADANDASANA (Balancing Stick Pose)

TECHNIQUE:

1. Stand with feet together. Raise arms from sides over the head bringing palms together in Namascar, elbows straight.

2. Step forward 2 feet with the right foot. Shift weight forward by bending at the waist and lower body with arms and head together as one unit. At the same time, lift the left leg, toe pointed, and knee locked, to the rear. The body, arms, and legs should now be parallel to the floor. Hold for 10 seconds.

3. Lowering the left leg, slowly step back to upright position, arms still extended above head. Change feet and step out 2 feet in front with the left leg and repeat pose. Hold 10 seconds.

4. Return to upright position. Lower arms to sides, palms down, and relax. Repeat.

BENEFITS: Firms and tightens hips, buttocks, and upper thighs. Enhances general circulation. Also helpful for strengthening abdomen and slimming upper arms.

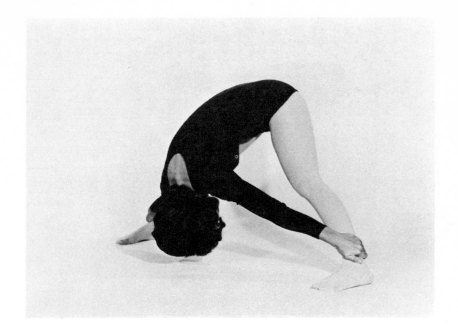

DANDAYAMANA-BIBHAKTAPADA-PASCHIMOTTHANASANA
(Standing Separate Leg Stretching Pose)

TECHNIQUE:

1.   Stand facing front. Step out to the right with feet 3 to 4 feet apart.

2.   Bend forward from the waist sliding hands down legs until fingers grip ankles, thumbs outside. Exhale and go down farther. Head should lightly touch the floor. *Knees are straight.*

3.   Hold 10 seconds with normal breathing throughout. Slowly straighten and bring feet together. Rest in position and repeat pose.

BENEFITS: Effective in reducing abdominal fat. Helps to relieve constipation. Enhances overall circulation.

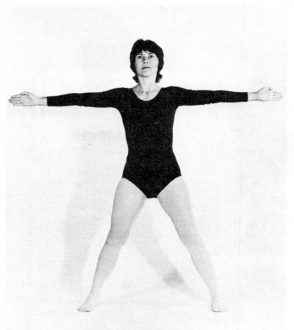 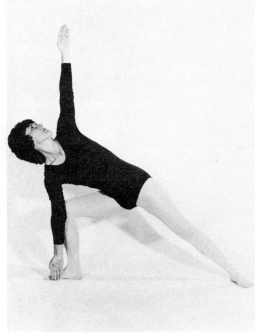

TRIKANASANA (Triangle Pose)

TECHNIQUE:

1. Stand erect. Raise arms sidewise above head until palms touch. Step out to the right about 3 feet. At the same time, lower arms until parallel to the floor.

2. Pivot your right foot to your right side as palms face forward. Slowly bend your right knee with left knee straight, raising face toward the ceiling, until arms are in one straight line and perpendicular to the floor. Your right elbow will be in front of your right knee. Chin may touch the deltoid muscle (shoulder).

3. Hold 10 seconds. Slowly straighten to standing position, pivot to the left and repeat on left side. Straighten to standing position, bring feet together, and lower arms to sides. Rest in position. Repeat pose.

BENEFITS: Especially effective in tightening upper thighs. Also slims hips and waistline.

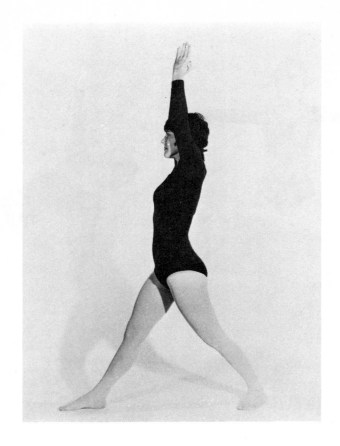

DANDAYAMANA-BIBHAKTAPADA-JANUSHIRASANA
(Standing Separate Leg Head to Knee Pose)

TECHNIQUE:

1. Stand erect. Raise arms sidewise above head until palms touch. Step out sidewise to the right about 3 feet. Pivot body to the right, arms above head.

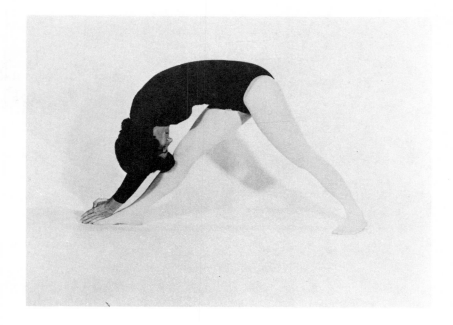

2. Bend forward directly over your right leg, arms and head together, until tips of your fingers touch your toes. Elbows and knees are straight.

3. Hold for 10 seconds. Return to standing position by raising up in line with the right leg.

4. Pivot to the left and go down. Touch toes of the left foot with fingertips and hold 10 seconds.

5. Straighten to standing position and pivot to the front.

6. Bring right foot back to left as you lower arms to the sides with palms down. Relax in standing position. Repeat pose.

BENEFITS: Slims abdomen and waistline. Tightens hips, buttocks, and upper thighs.

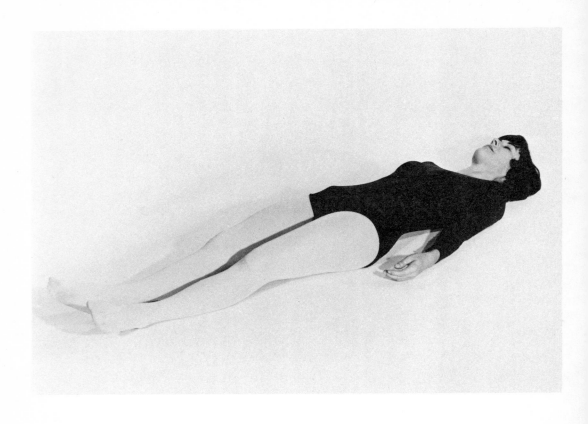

Sit-ups from Savasana

TECHNIQUE:

1. The proper way to get up from Savasana (Sponge Pose) after the birth of your baby is a sit-up. Lie down on your back in Savasana. When you are ready to rise, raise both arms above your head with hands together in Namascar. Inhale sharply through your nose, throw your hands over your head toward your toes and sit up.

2. Touch your toes twice and exhale twice through your mouth, making the sound, "HUH, HUH." This is the best way to rise from a prone position and is an exercise in itself.

BENEFITS: Excellent for strengthening and tightening the abdomen. Also firms upper arms.

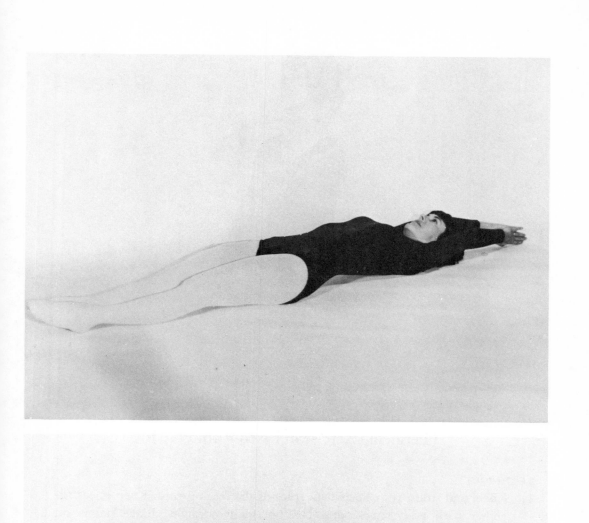

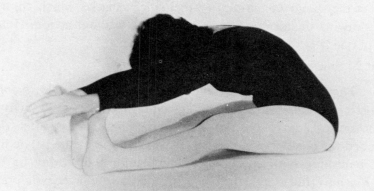

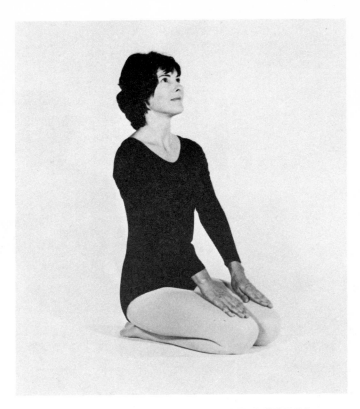

ASWINI-MUDRA IN VAJRASANA
(Perineal Exercise in Fixed Firm Pose)

TECHNIQUE:

1. Kneel and sit on your heels with soles of the feet upward. Keep knees to-gether with body, neck, and head perfectly straight. Place palms on knees.

2. Contract the sphincter muscles (the circular muscles which contract the anus) drawing them in as though to prevent a bowel action. Hold for a count of one beat; then relax for a count of one.

3. Repeat 25 times. Relax.

BENEFITS: *This is the most important exercise a woman can do before, during, and after pregnancy.* Practice of this Mudra increases elasticity of the pelvic floor muscles and helps to restore muscle function after delivery. Recommended for bladder symptoms due to relaxation of the pelvic muscles. Helpful in banishing both constipation and hemorrhoids. May be done in *Vipareeta-Karani* (Half-shoulder Stand) for increased efficiency in preventing or curing hemorrhoids. Also increases sexual proficiency and pleasure.

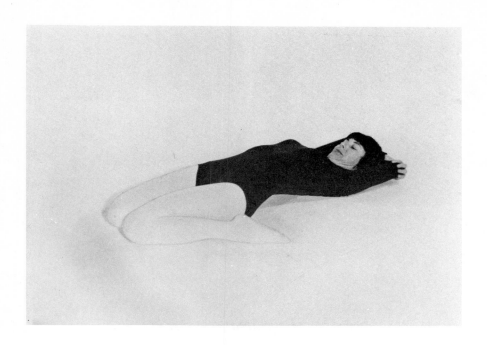

SUPTA-VAJRASANA (Full Fixed Firm Pose)

TECHNIQUE:
1. Sit on heels in Vajrasana (Fixed Firm Pose). Slide feet apart and sit between your legs with buttocks on the floor, legs touching hips.
2. Slowly let yourself back on your elbows until you are lying flat on the floor, knees together (if possible).
3. Tuck chin into notch between collarbone, grab elbows with hands over the head, and hold for 20 seconds. (The small of the back will bow up off the floor; this is natural.)
4. Slowly sit up using elbows and hands for support and lie down in Savasana. Rest for 20 seconds, sit up from Savasana, and repeat posture.

BENEFITS: Particularly effective in slimming thighs and firming calf muscles; also helpful in strengthening abdomen.

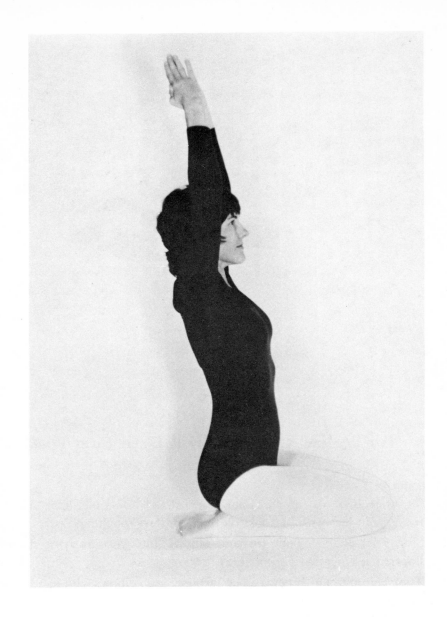

ARDHA-KURMASANA (Half Tortoise Pose)

TECHNIQUE:

1. Sit in Vajrasana (Fixed Firm Pose) with spine straight. Slowly raise arms sidewise above head until palms touch in Namascar.

HEALTHY PREGNANCY THE YOGA WAY

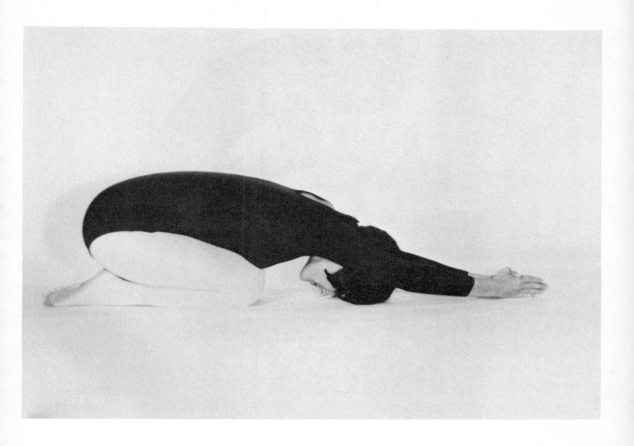

2. Moving arms and head together as one unit, stretch up and bend forward with elbows straight, until sides of palms touch the floor. Slide arms forward for maximum stretch without lifting buttocks from the heels and drop forehead to lightly graze the floor. (Elbows will be up off floor.)

3. Hold pose for 20 seconds. Slowly raise arms and head together to upright position. Lower hands sidewise. Rest in Savasana. Sit up and repeat pose.

BENEFITS: Strengthens abdominal muscles and removes fat in the abdomen and buttocks. Helps improve digestive power.

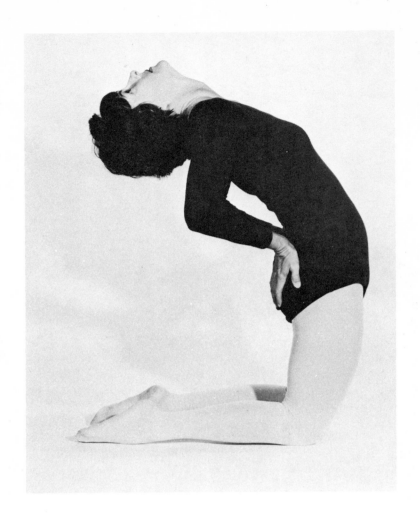

USTRASANA (Camel Pose)

TECHNIQUE:

1. Kneel with knees 6 inches apart, hands on buttocks. (Feet will also be 6 inches apart.)

2. Drop head back and slowly drop right hand to grip right heel with thumb outside. Then drop left hand to grip left heel in the same manner.

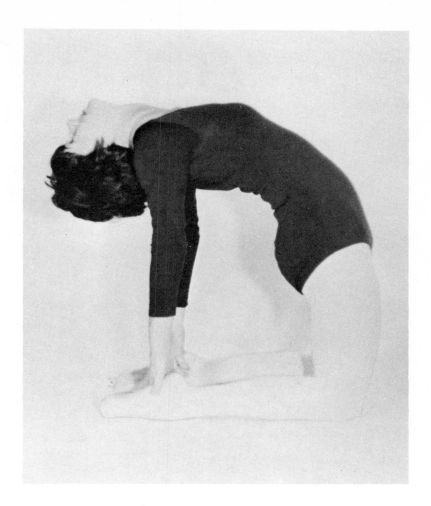

3. Push forward with the abdomen as much as possible and hold pose for 20 seconds. The inside of the back, head, arms, and legs should form a square.

4. Slowly come up with control. Lie down in Savasana and rest 20 seconds. Sit up and repeat posture.

BENEFITS: Ustrasana is an excellent posture for strengthening the lower back muscles and relieving backaches as the spine is compressed and shortened from 5 to 7 inches, greatly enhancing general circulation. Also stretches and firms the abdomen and waistline. This posture should always be followed by the reverse pose, Sasangasana (Rabbit Pose).

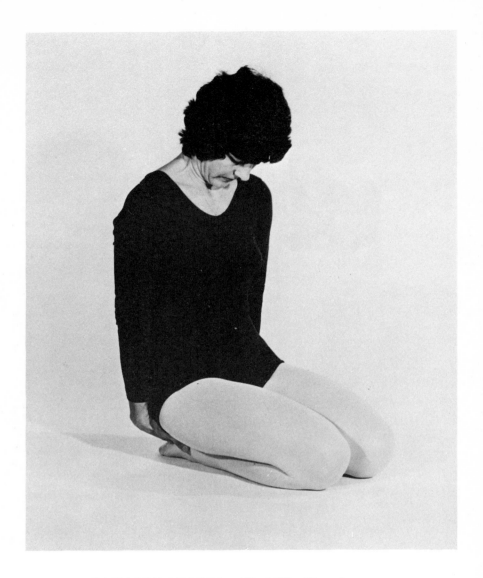

SASANGASANA (Rabbit Pose)

TECHNIQUE:

1. Sit in Vajrasana (Fixed Firm Pose). Bend forward a little and catch hold of both heels with the palms.

2. Bend forward holding both heels firmly, thumbs outside, until the forehead touches the knees. Place the center of the head lightly on the floor and press the throat with the chin. Push the back and buttocks forward, bowing up the back without changing the position of the head and knees, until the arms become straight.

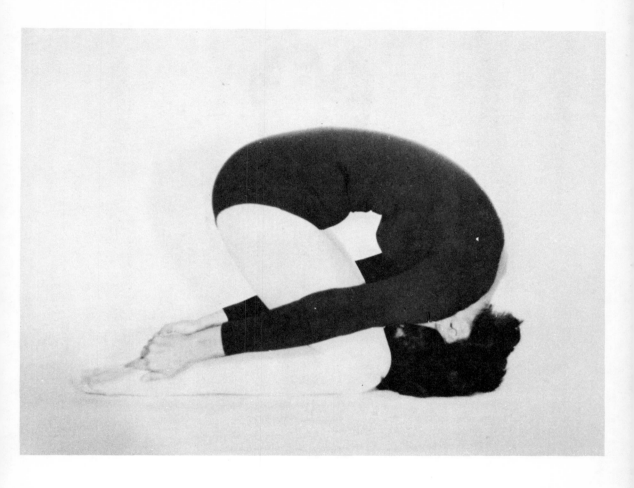

3. Eyes remain open to avoid dizziness. Hold for 20 seconds, normal breathing throughout.

4. *Slowly* return to upright position, retaining grip on the heels until erect. Relax in Savasana, sit up, and repeat pose.

BENEFITS: Sasangasana makes the spine flexible by exercising and relaxing the joints. The spine will be stretched and lengthened from 5 to 7 inches while performing this Asana. This is the best possible stretching exercise for the spine. Also excellent for toning the abdomen. Sasangasana is the reverse posture for Ustrasana (Camel Pose).

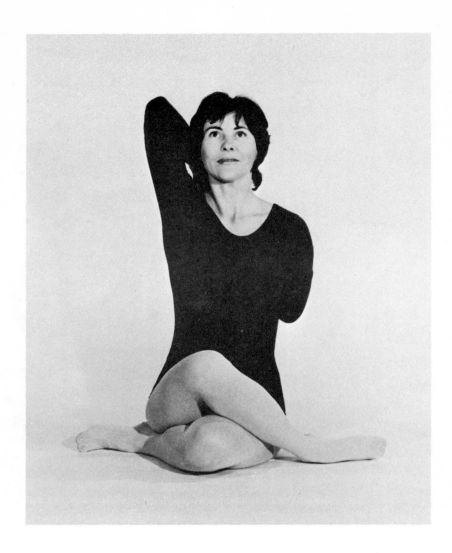

GOMUKHASANA (Cow Face Pose)

TECHNIQUE:

1. Place left heel against the right buttock and right heel against the left buttock, so that the two knees are exactly above one another.

2. With the right hand, grasp the three center fingers of the left hand behind the back. The right elbow will point upward. Spine is straight.

HEALTHY PREGNANCY THE YOGA WAY

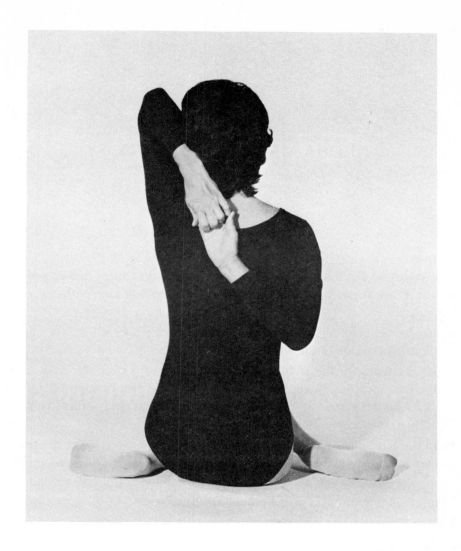

3. Hold for 20 seconds. Change sides, alternating position of the legs and arms; when the right knee is on top of the left knee, the right elbow will point upward and vice versa. Hold for 20 seconds. Relax in Savasana. Sit up and repeat posture.

BENEFITS: Firms the breasts and upper arms. Tightens upper thighs, hips, and buttocks. Relieves backache.

NOTE: Beginners may not be able to grip hands immediately. This will improve with daily practice.

ARDHA-MATSYENDRASANA
(Spine Twisting Pose)

TECHNIQUE:

1. Sit straight on the buttocks with legs stretched out in front and closed together. Place the left heel against the right buttock underneath the right leg.

2. Bring the right leg over the left thigh and place the sole of the foot flat on the floor by the side of the left thigh.

3. Twist the trunk to the right and bring the left arm over the right knee with elbow touching the calf and the inside of the arm facing out. (Keep the left shoulder and the right knee pressed against each other with the right thigh pressing against the abdomen.)

4. Hold the left knee by the left palm and at the same time, twist the trunk farther to the right, looking over your right shoulder. Try to touch the inner side of the upper left thigh with your right hand. Hold 20 seconds.

5. Change sides and repeat pose holding for 20 seconds.

6. Rest in Savasana, sit up, and repeat posture.

BENEFITS: Increases elasticity of the spine and massages the abdomen and internal organs. Enhances general circulation. An aid to reducing excess weight and slimming the waistline.

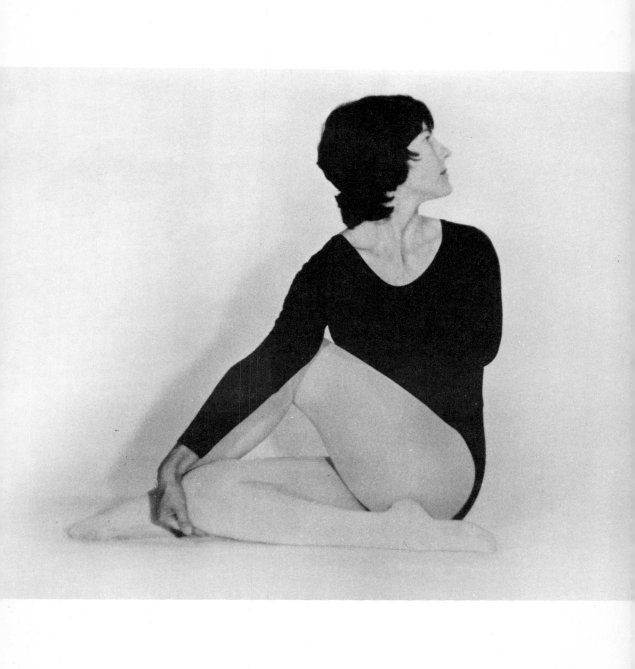

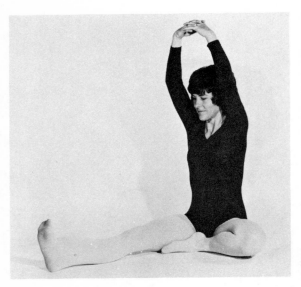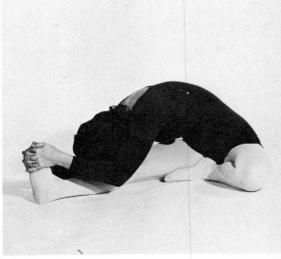

JANUSHIRASANA WITH PASCHIMOTTHANASANA
(Sitting Head to Knee Pose
with Stretching Posture)

TECHNIQUE:

1. Sit on the floor with both legs stretched out in front. Draw in the left leg and place the left heel at the beginning of the right thigh with the left sole against the inner side of the right thigh. Be sure to keep the right leg fully stretched.

2. Interlock fingers of both hands, inhale and raise arms above head. Exhale and grasp the toes of the right foot with both hands, bending forward until the forehead touches the right knee. Hold for 10 seconds.

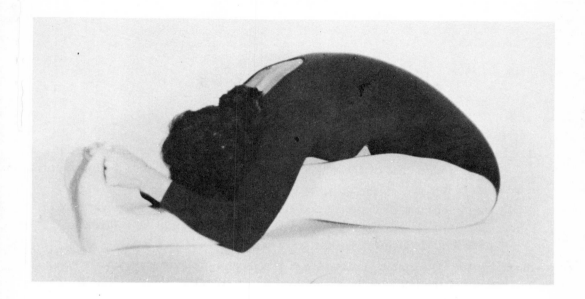

3. Change sides, grasping the toes of the left foot and touching the forehead to the left knee. Hold for 10 seconds.

4. Lie back in Savasana. Raise both arms over the head, pressing the ears, inhale, and sit up. Exhale and bend forward until palms reach the toes. Hold the respective big toes by the first two fingers of each hand and continue to bend the trunk slowly forward until the forehead touches the knees and the elbows touch the floor. (Knees are not bent; legs remain flat on the floor.)

5. Hold for 20 seconds. Raise up and lie down in Savasana. Rest, sit up, and repeat posture.

BENEFITS: Excellent for reducing abdominal fat. Helps to reduce flatulence.

NOTE: Beginners are allowed to bend their knees as it may be impossible to keep the legs perfectly straight at the outset. Improvement will be noticed each time the Asana is performed.

BHUJANGASANA (Cobra Pose)

TECHNIQUE:

1. Lie face down on the floor. Place palms on the floor underneath the shoulders with tips of the fingers pointing forward and just below the shoulder line.

2. Keeping legs together, inhale and raise the chest, looking up toward the ceiling until elbows form a 90° angle. Shoulders should be relaxed and elbows should touch sides of the body at all times.

3. Hold for 20 seconds. You will feel pressure on your lower back as you are lifting the body by the strength of the spine rather then pushing it up with the arms.

4. Slowly lower to prone position and relax on your stomach. Repeat posture.

BENEFITS: Helps prevent lower backache and makes the spine flexible. Improves posture. This Asana is very beneficial for any kind of menstrual troubles as the blood circulation through the ovaries and surroundings, including the lumbar vertebra, is greatly increased.

NOTE: The four Asanas of the Cobra Series (Bhujangasana, Salabhasana, Poorna-Salabhasana and Dhanurasana) should be performed together as a series and are among the most beneficial for women.

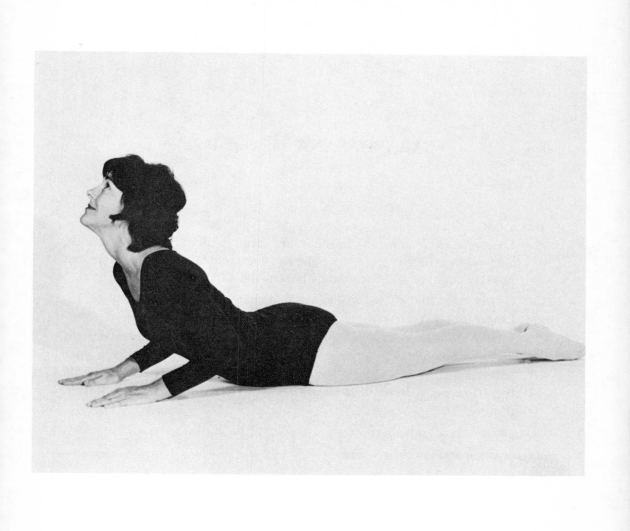

SALABHASANA (Locust Pose)

TECHNIQUE:

1. Lie prone with chin on the floor and arms underneath the abdomen, palms down. Slowly raise the right leg, toe pointed, to a 45° angle and hold for count of 10. Knee should be straight. Lower leg and relax.

2. Slowly raise the left leg in the same manner and hold for count of 10. Lower leg and relax.

3. Inhale and raise both legs together as far as possible with knees straight and toes pointed. As you raise your legs, press the floor hard with your palms; this acts as a natural lever and helps to assume the posture. Hold for 10 seconds, lower legs slowly and with control, and relax. Repeat posture.

BENEFITS: Especially good for firming buttocks and hips. Helps eliminate constipation and lower backache.

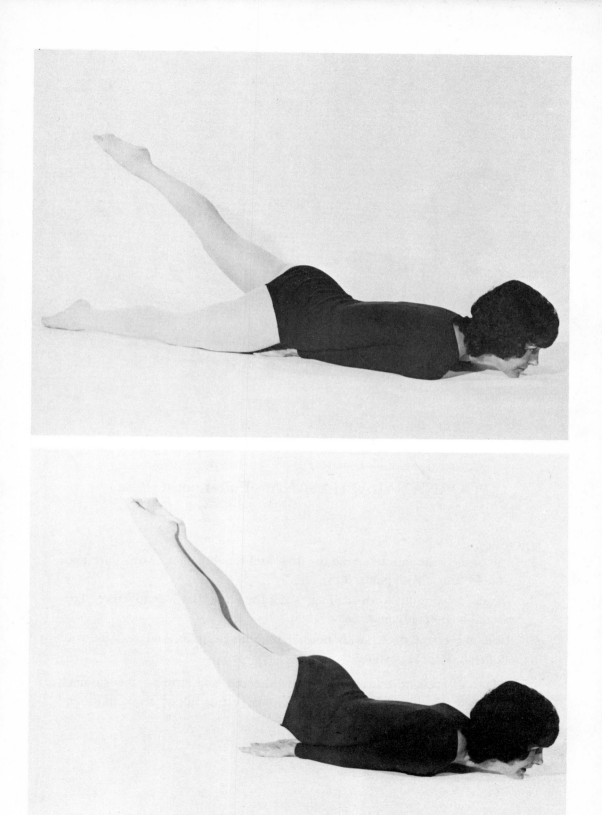

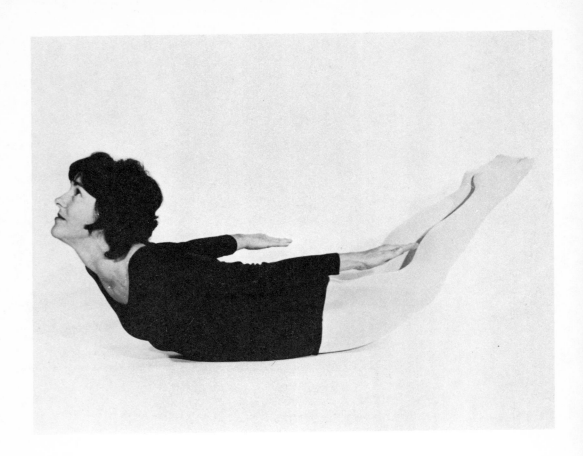

POORNA-SALABHASANA (Full Locust Pose)

TECHNIQUE:

1. Lie prone with chin touching the floor and legs together. Arms flare back at a 45° angle with palms down.

2. Inhale, looking up to the ceiling, and raise chest and legs together. Toes should be pointed and knees straight.

3. Hold for count of 10 with normal breathing. Relax and rest on your stomach. Repeat posture.

BENEFITS: Excellent exercise for strengthening and firming the stomach muscles. Aids in eliminating lower back pain. Firms upper arms, hips, and thighs.

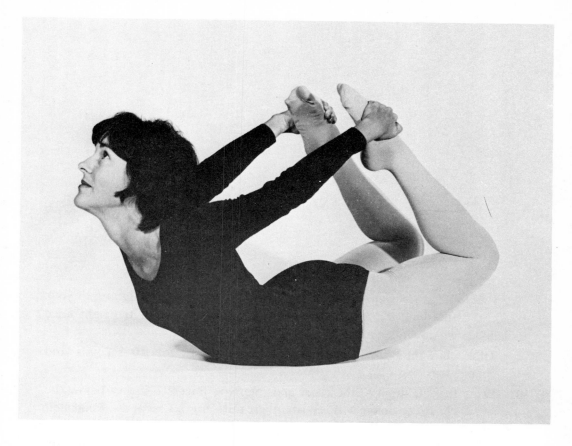

DHANURASANA (Bow Pose)

TECHNIQUE:

1. Lie face down with legs stretched straight out but slightly apart, arms parallel to the sides, and chin touching the floor.

2. Bend the legs and grip the ankles with both hands, thumbs outside. Knees should be in line with the shoulders.

3. Look up toward the ceiling, raise the chest, and kick back and up with toes pointed. Do not jerk; the movement should be slow and smooth.

4. Hold position for 10 seconds. Slowly relax and rest in face down pose. Repeat posture.

BENEFITS: Reduces abdominal fat and improves abdominal blood circulation. Makes the spine flexible and helps to cure constipation. This pose is very energizing and definitely improves vitality.

NOTE: This Asana must be avoided by those with high blood pressure.

PAVANAMUKTASANA (Gas Removing Pose)

TECHNIQUE:

1. Lie down in Savasana. Bend the right leg and bring your thigh up to your chest. Interlock the fingers of both hands 2 inches below the right knee and press down, keeping elbows close to the sides.

2. Tuck chin into notch between collarbone. Hold for 20 seconds and change legs.

3. Bring the left thigh to the chest and interlock fingers 2 inches below the left knee. Press down with constant pressure for 20 seconds. Relax left leg.

4. Bring both legs up together and grab elbows over the knees with both hands. Hold tightly, pressing both thighs against the chest, for 20 seconds. Relax legs and rest in Savasana. Repeat posture.

BENEFITS: As the name implies, this Asana is effective for removing gas from the intestines. Also reduces abdominal fat and increases flexibility of the knees and hips.

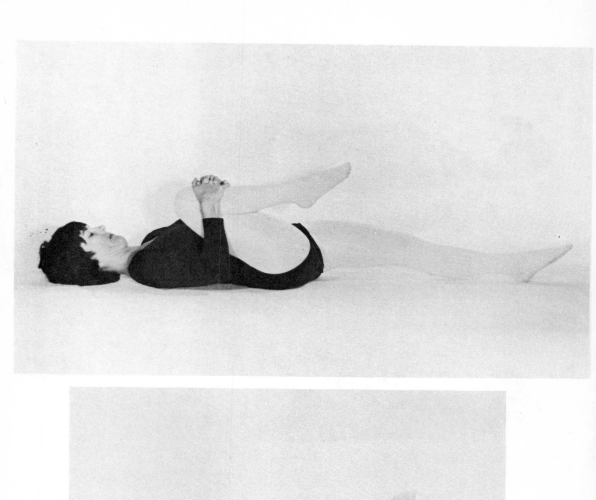

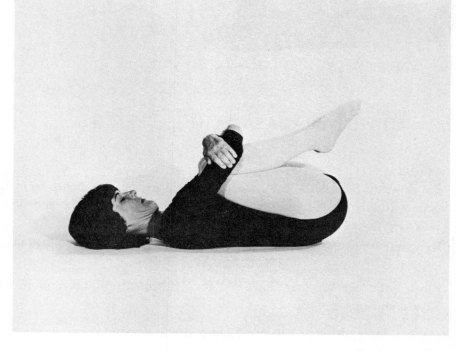

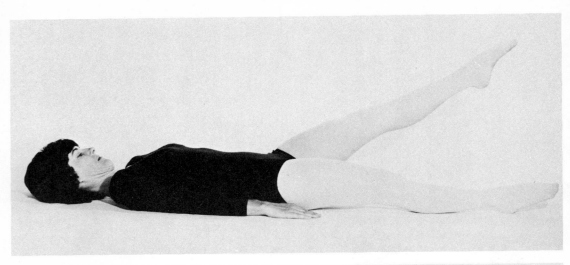

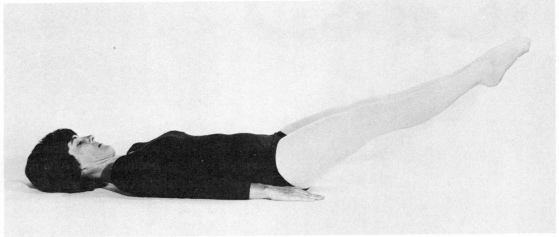

UTTHITA-PADASANA (Leg Lifting Pose)

TECHNIQUE:

1. Lie down in Savasana. Raise the right leg up about 10 inches from the floor with toe pointed and knee locked. Hold for count of 10 and slowly lower leg.

2. Raise left leg in the same manner and hold for count of 10. Slowly lower left leg.

3. Raise both legs together and hold for 10 seconds. Relax and rest in Savasana. Repeat pose.

BENEFITS: Strengthens and firms abdominal muscles and removes gas from intestines. Also strengthens the legs.

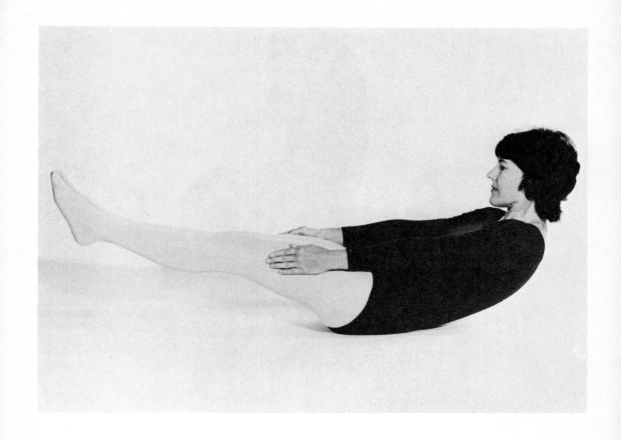

THE BOAT (Head and Leg Lifting Pose)

TECHNIQUE:

1. Lie down in Savasana. Inhale and raise your head and chest off the floor as you raise both legs together, toes pointed. Arms will touch the sides of the body and slide down to touch the outside thighs as you come up. Both head and feet should be even and about 2 feet from the floor.

2. Hold for 10 seconds. Relax, rest in Savasana and repeat pose.

BENEFITS: Excellent for firming the abdomen and strengthening abdominal muscles and upper thighs.

NOTE: Do not be alarmed if your stomach muscles tremble. This simply means they are weak and need strengthening.

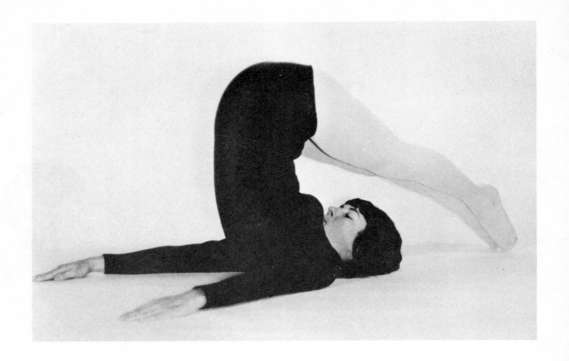

HALASANA (Plough Pose)

TECHNIQUE:

1. Lie in Savasana with palms pressing down against the floor.
2. Slowly and steadily raise legs from the floor keeping them straight and together. Raise them over the head until toes touch the floor. Knees remain straight. Palms continue to press firmly against the floor to give a thrust to the lifting movement and to keep the balance. Chin will press tightly against the chest.
3. Hold position for 20 seconds. Return to Savasana slowly and with control. Relax. May repeat a second time.

BENEFITS: Reduces fat on abdomen. Makes the spine flexible and helps to banish backache and constipation. Firms stomach, hips, and legs. Also beneficial for upper arms.

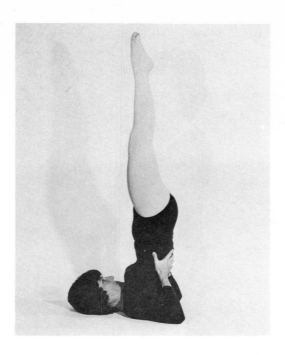

SARVANGASANA (Shoulder Stand)

TECHNIQUE:

1. Lie down in Savasana. Bring your knees to your chest and slowly raise your hips off the floor.

2. Place your hands in the small of the back with elbows resting on the floor and slowly straighten your legs with toes pointed up toward the ceiling. Weight is centered on the shoulders and back of the neck. Chin is pressed tightly to the chest in a chin lock. Legs should be as straight as possible.

3. Hold posture for 20 seconds. Slowly relax by dropping knees to forehead, bending the spine and rolling smoothly back into Savasana, one vertebra at a time. Rest in Savasana. You may repeat pose a second time if desired.

BENEFITS: This is a superb Yogasana and one of the most important postures to practice. It keeps the body youthful and enhances overall circulation. Additionally, it is helpful in weight control and in delaying aging. Helps restore sagging tissues and the displacement of vital organs by counteracting the force of gravity. Helps relieve the symptoms of varicose veins. Extremely important as a post-natal exercise for new mothers!

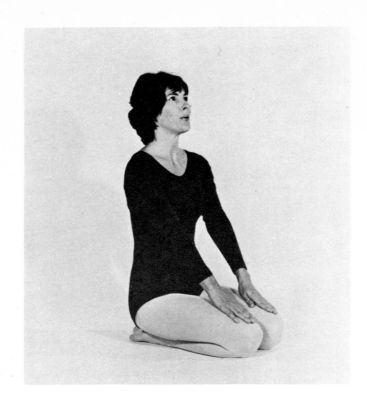

KAPALBHATI IN VAJRASANA
(Blowing in Fixed Firm Pose)

TECHNIQUE:

1. Sit in Vajrasana (Fixed Firm Pose) with hands resting on knees. Eyes concentrate on one spot in the distance.

2. Blow out sharply through pursed lips as though to blow out a candle. At the same time, contract the stomach by an inward jerk of the abdomen.

3. Count rythmically to 100 giving each breath one count, approximately one expulsion per second. Attention should be focused on maintaining rhythmic diaphragmatic action with emphasis on exhalation.

4. Rest in Savasana from 3 to 10 minutes and relax completely.

BENEFITS: This recharging breath is an energizing technique as well as a fine exercise for strengthening abdominal muscles. Kapalbhati stimulates all the tissues of the body. Always end your exercise period with Kapalbhati followed by Savasana.

NOTE: Take care not to hyperventilate when doing Kapalbhati. If hands and feet start to tingle or vision is affected, stop immediately and relax in Savasana.

8

A NEW YOU
THROUGH YOGA !

Exercise and Energize

Hatha Yoga is the most complete exercise system devised as it works on the entire being. Yoga improves a person mentally by building will power and patience, physically by improving strength, flexibility, and balance, and emotionally by inducing serenity, tranquility, and peace of mind. A well-balanced person is one who is able to integrate these three levels—the mental, the physical, and the spiritual—and it is the culmination of the first two that leads to the third. With a healthy body comes a healthy mind, and the body must be in top condition before the mind can follow. That is why in India, the first step on the ladder to Enlightenment or Raja Yoga begins with Hatha Yoga.

Regular practice of Yoga also improves and firms the figure by reducing fat and trimming inches, improves the skin and complexion by increasing the circulation, and revitalizes the body by self-energization techniques. Yoga also aims to improve the circulatory, abdominal, and nervous systems, from which many medical problems stem.

Through Yogasanas and Pranayama techniques, the body is so energized that the need for rest and sleep is naturally diminished. Many people who practice Yoga report a dramatic change in their sleeping habits, stating that they just don't seem to need as much sleep as before. Practicing yogis sleep but a few hours a night and many eat but one full meal a day, drawing the majority of their life energy or Prana from the air they breathe. Through the deep relaxation experienced through Yoga, the body is revitalized, a lighter diet becomes adequate, and the need for long hours of sleep is reduced.

Flab . . . It Doesn't Have to Be!

Flab is caused by lack of muscle tone resulting from insufficient exercise, stretched tissues, or excessive weight gain. However, people who are not overweight may also suffer from flab. Daily exercise is the way to tighten and firm muscles that have become stretched and slack from pregnancy or lack of exercise. Yoga tightens and firms the figure as it trims inches, but for best results it must be practiced *every day*. It is this daily effort that makes the difference between an effective exercise program and an ineffective one; a sporadic effort based on good intentions does not produce results. Yoga is self-perpetuating in that the very practice of the Yogasanas builds the will power and patience necessary to stick with any program of exercise. Work at your own Yoga program with daily discipline and at your own speed. It is better to devote 10 or 20 minutes a day, every day on a regular basis, than it is to complete 1½ hours of Yoga once a week. Yoga should become an integral part of your life and as much a daily habit as eating or sleeping.

Yogasanas are unsurpassed for stretching and activating all the muscles in your body in a way that no other exercise can. Jogging uses 7 per cent of your muscle groups, swimming uses 10 per cent, and bicycling 12 per cent, but with a fell session of Yoga, you exercise 100 per cent of your muscle groups. A complete program of Yoga reaches every muscle, organ, fiber, and nerve. Yogasanas are the only exercises that attack the inner upper thighs, a favorite place for flab to accumulate. If you are bothered by particular areas of flab, such as the back-hip or under-arm area, concentrate on the spot Asanas recommended for these parts of the body and practice them two or three times a day apart from your regular exercise session.

Weight Gain and Excess Poundage

Most obstetricians agree that a woman may expect to gain about twenty-five pounds during her pregnancy if she weighed close to the normal average for her height and build in the beginning. Gaining too much weight during pregnancy is to be avoided as it can be associated with severe problems such as high blood pressure, toxemia, and a difficult delivery. Too small a weight gain can be harmful to the child, so pregnancy is definitely not the time to go on a diet.

A new mother frequently discovers after delivery that she has added a few pounds and inches. Yoga offers a natural way of weight regulation that easily becomes an enjoyable part of your life. Daily practice of a complete set of Yogasanas offers the most efficient exercise possible for weight control. However, while exercise can firm and tone your body, exercise alone cannot eliminate excess weight gain, and must go hand in hand with a sensible diet based on nutritious and healthful foods. A yogic diet composed of natural life-force foods is often sufficient, but if you have a severe weight problem, consult your doctor for a proper diet to follow and don't experiment with drugs or dietary fads.

Eliminate pastries and sweets, rich meals, and fried foods when trying to lose weight and concentrate on a diet of fresh fruits and vegetables, skim milk and milk products, eggs, meat, and fish, if desired, and plenty of fruit juices and water. Sufficient fluids are a must for the nursing mother and are also important in keeping the system clear. If you are a nursing mother, you must be particularly careful to include enough of the nutritional needs to supply your baby with the quantity and quality of milk he requires. The same Yoga foods that were helpful in your pre-natal diet are the foods that can help you slim down and stay slim after baby arrives.

STAY AWAY FROM:

pastries, cakes, and pies

ice cream and puddings

potato chips and salted nuts

bacon, sausages, and franks

chocolate

sour cream (substitute yogurt)

canned fruits, vegetables, and soups

carbonated drinks

pickles and olives

macaroni and spaghetti

fried foods

rich sauces and gravies

mayonnaise

alcohol

TV dinners

EAT PLENTY OF:

fresh fruits and vegetables

nuts and seeds (unsalted)

skim milk or low-fat milk

milk products such as cheese, cottage
    cheese, yogurt, and buttermilk

lean meats, poultry, and fish in
    moderate amounts

whole-grain rice, breads, and cereals

fresh herbs and herb teas

A limited diet is not necessarily a dull diet. Use your imagination to conjure up menus and dishes that are tantalizing to the eye and the taste buds. Salads can be endlessly improvised depending upon what is fresh and in season. If you do "fall off the wagon," enjoy it and climb right back on again!

Self-discipline Can Work Miracles

Discipline is very much needed during pregnancy, not only for itself but in preparation for the discipline needed in caring for a new baby. You may skip a day of exercise if you choose, but a baby must be taken care of *every* day. The patience and self-discipline obtained through regular Yoga practice during pregnancy is invaluable after the baby arrives.

Self-discipline is a necessary part of achieving your goals, but first you must determine exactly what it is that you wish to accomplish. Verbalize your aims and define your goals as clearly as you can. Write them down in complete detail, being as specific and as thorough as possible. Next, decide exactly what you can do to realize your goals, and write this down too, as precisely as you can. Now, sit quietly for a few moments and close your eyes; on the screen of your imagination, see yourself as you are today, honestly, perhaps a bit heavier than you'd like, with an unwelcome bit of flab here or there. Visualize yourself clearly; then erase your screen. Now, see yourself as you would *like* to appear, slim, trim, and vibrating with health and vitality. Picture your hair, your clothes, and shoes, and visualize every detail *exactly* as you would like it. See yourself smiling and happy, doing the things you would like to do, living up to your highest ambitions. Visualize as vividly as possible and hold the image until it "sets" and becomes real to you. This is the mental image you have constructed as your goal; hold this image in your mind and refer to it often during the day. Actually *see* yourself as looking this way and *know* that it will come to pass.

Self-discipline is, simply stated, deciding exactly what you must do to accomplish your goals, and then doing it. Yoga helps to develop the purposeful concentration, patience, and will power necessary to realize your goals, whatever they may be!

A POST - NATAL POSTSCRIPT

Natural Family Planning . . .
The Ovulation Method

A little known but highly effective natural method of birth control is now available which enables all future pregnancies to be planned. Called the Ovulation Method, it is a way of birth control completely free from pills, drugs, appliances, or other artificial and sometimes dangerous means of prevention. Developed by two Australian physicians, the Ovulation Method is a distinct method to be used alone and is a natural and completely harmless means of control. It does not require regularity of the cycles, is simple to understand, and can be taught by one woman to another. Although there is no basic contradiction between the various natural means of birth control, the Rhythm Method or Calendar Method and the Temperature Method are sometimes inaccurate, while the Ovulation Method is 100 per cent accurate if properly applied. The Ovulation Method is based on the pattern of cervical mucus which has been demonstrated to reflect the hormonal events that accompany ovulation and has been successfully taught to women around the world, including women in primitive tribes and even blind women. All women can learn to recognize the symptoms of monthly ovulation and apply this method. *Natural Family Planning, The Ovulation Method* by John J. Billings, M.D., is available through your gynecologist or through The Liturgical Press, Collegeville, Minnesota.